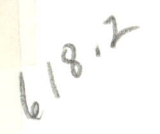

Etta "Granny" Nichols—Last Of The Old-Timey Midwives

By

Sharon Smith-Ledford

Copyright © 1998 Sharon Smith-Ledford
All Rights Reserved

No part of this book may be reproduced or transmitted in any form or by any means, electronic, mechanical, including photocopying, recording, or by any information storage and retrieval system, except in the case of reviews, without the express written permission of the publisher, except where permitted by law.

Library of Congress Catalog Number 97-76585

ISBN Number 1-57087-363-1

Professional Press
Chapel Hill, NC 27515-4371

Manufactured in the United States of America
00 99 98   10 9 8 7 6 5 4 3 2 1

Acknowledgments

I wish to express my deepest appreciation to all my family members for sharing their stories with me concerning my grandmother, Etta Nichols. I also want to thank all the women who answered my newspaper ad when I was searching for women to interview whom Etta had performed deliveries for, and allowing me to use their stories in my book.

A special thanks goes to Furman Grigsby, and Loiree Grigsby Collins for providing information contained in "Ancestral History" and "Life Growing Up."

To Traci Smith, Darren Burgin, Sheri Burgin Stinnett, and Felicia Guillot Rogers, thanks so much for your helpful assistance in the preparation of my manuscript.

To my sisters, Lynda and Venida, thank you for <u>all</u> your support.

I want to thank all the newspapers for doing such a wonderful job on their interviews with my grandmother, and for giving me permission to use these articles in my book.

To Michael Sylva and Joan Beaver, thank you for allowing me to use your photos and drawings in my book.

My family and I wish to extend our deepest and warmest appreciation to all the nurses from Smoky Mountain Home Health who provided such wonderful care for our loved one, Etta Nichols.

*In Memory Of
My Loving Grandmother*

Carrie Etta Nichols

Dedicated To:

My Mother, Belle Nichols Smith
and
My Daughter, Tiffany Alise Smith

A Message From The Author

To write about my grandmother's life story is truly an honor. I hope I have done her justice. If so, I have no doubt the reader will be inspired, and impressed with the life she led.

It is not my intent to become rich from the sale of this book, but to introduce Etta Nichols into the lives of as many people as possible. She devoted her life to helping others with no expectation of payment from her patients. When she did receive payment, she never charged more than $15.00 for a delivery, although a few nice people made her accept more.

As a tribute to my loving grandmother, Etta Nichols, I am charging only $15.00 each for the first printing of the soft covered books. This price will barely cover the expenses I have incurred while preparing this book, but I want to make it as low in cost as possible for my readers so more people can afford to purchase it and enrich their lives through her example.

Enjoy the story...you are about to meet a truly incredible person!!!

List Of Family Characters

Gilliland, John Thomas	Husband of June Nichols
Gilliland, June Nichols	Second child of Harrison and Etta Nichols
Gilliland, Geraldine	First child of John and June Gilliland
Gilliland, Virginia Ann	Second child of John and June Gilliland
Gilliland, Tommy	Third child of John and June Gilliland
Gilliland, Johnnie Sue	Fourth child of John and June Gilliland
Grigsby, J. B., Dr.	Etta Grigsby Nichols' Grandfather
Grigsby, John Lewis	Etta Grigsby Nichols' Father
Grigsby, Nova Turner	Etta Grigsby Nichols' Mother
Grigsby, Lewis	First child of John Lewis and Nova Grigsby
Grigsby, Margaret Carrie Etta	Second child of John Lewis and Nova Grigsby
Grigsby, Waitsel	Third child of John Lewis and Nova Grigsby

Grigsby, Paul	Fourth child of John Lewis and Nova Grigsby
Grigsby, Alverta	Fifth child of John Lewis and Nova Grigsby
Grigsby, Willie (Bill)	Sixth child of John Lewis and Nova Grigsby
Grigsby, Creed	Seventh child of John Lewis and Nova Grigsby
Grigsby, Lurlie	Eighth child of John Lewis and Nova Grigsby
Grigsby, John Louis (J. L.)	Ninth child of John Lewis and Nova Grigsby
Grigsby, Furman	Tenth child of John Lewis and Nova Grigsby
Grigsby, Loiree Smith	Wife of J. L. Grigsby, sister to Floyd J. Smith
Grigsby, Dianne	First born child of J. L. and Loiree Grigsby
Grigsby, Michael	Second child of J. L. and Loiree Grigsby
Jones, Richard (Dick)	Husband of Emily Nichols
Jones, Emily Nichols	First child of Harrison and Etta Nichols
Jones, Valerie	First child of Dick and Emily Jones
Jones, Sandra	Second child of Dick and Emily Jones

Jones, Darrell	Third child of Dick and Emily Jones
Jones, Debbie	Fourth child of Dick and Emily Jones
Nichols, James Harrison	Husband of Etta Grigsby
Nichols, Etta "Granny"	Famous First Lady of Del Rio
Nichols, Emily	First child of Harrison and Etta Nichols
Nichols, June	Second child of Harrison and Etta Nichols
Nichols, Jasper Lewis (Jack)	Third child of Harrison and Etta Nichols
Nichols, Margaret Belle	Fourth child of Harrison and Etta Nichols
Nichols, Juanita Finchum	Wife of Jack Nichols
Nichols, Susan	First child of Jack and Juanita Nichols
Nichols, James Lewis (Jimmy)	Second child of Jack and Juanita Nichols
Smith, Floyd Jay	Husband of Belle Nichols
Smith, Belle Nichols	Fourth child of Harrison and Etta Nichols
Smith, Floyd Ray	First child of Floyd and Belle Smith
Smith, Lynda Carol	Second child of Floyd and Belle Smith

Smith, Venida Ellen   Third child of Floyd and Belle Smith

Smith, Sharon Kay   Fourth child of Floyd and Belle Smith

Contents

PROLOGUE xii

ANCESTRAL HISTORY xvii

LIST OF ARTICLES AND INTERVIEWS ETTA
NICHOLS APPEARED IN xxvi

PART I   LIFE GROWING UP 1

PART II   MARRIED LIFE 23

PART III   THE BIRTH OF A NEW MIDWIFE 51

PART IV   O SWEET GRANDMOTHER 81

PART V   MIDDLE AGED AND COUNTING 133

PART VI   BECOMING A LIVING LEGEND 163

PART VII   HEAVEN AWAITS 232

MORE PHOTOS 255

Prologue

On November 18, 1994, Belle Smith, the youngest of Carrie Etta Nichols' four children, was awakened around 3 A.M. by her mother. "She was singing the prettiest song, and she spoke her words so clearly. It was almost as if she knew something was about to happen," Belle told her children the following day. Later that day Etta had a stroke, leaving her throat paralyzed. The nurse from the home health agency said Etta would probably do well to live another week. She was no longer able to eat or drink because the stroke prevented her from swallowing.

The following week was a true test of faith for the family of Margaret Carrie Etta Grigsby Nichols...known as "Granny Nichols" to most people who knew her.

Exactly one week later, on Friday, November 25, 1994, Etta lay in her twin-size hospital bed between clean white sheets and a pale blue blanket which covered her frail, withered body. Her waist-length brown-and-gray hair lay plaited in one large strand by her side. It shimmered in the illuminating sunlight which beamed through the windows opposite her bed. Snow-white strands framed her face, creating a softness around her beautiful blue eyes which one only earns through graciousness. Her bed was placed in the master bedroom of Belle's nine-room house. A full-size antique bed with a white headboard occupied the space to the left of Etta where Belle slept, while the blue wall on her right held a four-space picture frame containing pictures of Belle's four children, Etta's grandchildren. Etta often had stared at the pictures on the wall during her two previous years of being bedfast there. She told any visitors, "That's my kids up there." There was Floyd Ray, the oldest, then Lynda, Venida, and Sharon. She did not realize they were not her children, but her grandchildren.

A white antique chest stood in the room toward the foot of Etta's bed; a matching dresser sat along the right wall at the foot of Belle's bed. A beautiful blue water pitcher and basin rested on top of the chest while the dresser held family pictures and other odds and ends. On Belle's headboard were two small reading lamps, and a stuffed koala bear from Australia which Floyd Ray had sent to his mother during his tour in Vietnam. The Holy Bible lay alongside the Sunday school lesson for the following Sunday's church service, which Belle studied while she rested in her bed each night.

Etta seemed quite content to have never been out of the bed for over two years, but she never was one to complain about anything. She accepted life the way God sent it to her, and she made the most of it.

Etta had four children. Only three of her children were still alive: June Gilliland, Jack Nichols, and Belle Smith. Her first child, Emily Jones, died on February 2, 1971, at the Baptist Hospital in Knoxville, Tennessee. She suffered a brain hemorrhage 10 days after a stroke.

June had been staying with Belle for a few days so she could help Belle with their mother, and to be close to Etta during the time she had left.

On this day, Belle decided she needed to go to Newport to get some medicine for her mother, and to pick up some items at the grocery store. She and her grandson, Darren Burgin, left the house around 10 A.M. They had not been gone long when Venida went to check on her grandmother. Venida noticed Etta's hands were turning blue. She had been told by the nurse, who had been there only a couple of hours earlier, that this was one of the signs to look for to know that death was near. Venida went into the kitchen to call her Uncle Jack, who lived in the peaceful, isolated hollow directly behind Belle's house. Venida informed him, "I think it's time." She waited for Jack to arrive before telling her Aunt June, who was in the kitchen washing dishes. Jack was there in a matter of minutes. Venida also called her sister, Lynda Burgin, and Lynda's husband, Edd, to come to the house. They also lived close by.

Felicia, Venida's daughter, stood on the right side of her great-grandmother's bed holding her frail, wrinkled hand in hers. Venida, Lynda, and Edd stood at the foot of the bed, while June and Jack stood on the left side of the bed—all waiting for the inevitable. June bent over the cold, silver bedside rails which stretched along the side of the bed and kissed her mother on the forehead. "I love you, Mother," were the last words June said to her.

Etta opened her eyes wide as she looked up at her daughter and her only son standing over her.

"I think she knows you," Felicia said to June.

"No, Honey. She don't know," responded Jack.

Etta closed her eyes and released her last breath at the age of ninety-seven.

"I'll bet angels are in this room right now," proclaimed Venida.

It was 10:45 A.M. when Sharon received the shattering news while working at her job in Morristown. "Sharon, Mamaw just died," came Venida's quavering voice over the phone. Venida gave Sharon, her sister, the details that had just unfolded. Sharon's eyes filled with tears as she listened. No one could have loved their grandmother more than she did.

Belle and Darren returned home about 30 minutes after Etta's passing. Edd met Belle outside as she approached the front door. "She's gone," Edd said sympathetically.

Belle's eyes opened widely in astonishment. "Oh, she is?" asked Belle in a shocked tone. (It was later discussed among the family members how God must have intended for Belle to be gone when her mother passed away, for she had not left her side for weeks until this very morning at this very hour. He must have known she would not have been able to handle watching her mother take her last breath.)

Belle entered the bedroom she had shared with her mother for the past two years. There she released the tears she had been desperately trying to hold back as she said her final good-bye to her beloved mother.

Carrie Etta Nichols felt herself being released from the worn and wrinkled body her spirit had inhabited for the past 97 years. She felt light and totally free as her spirit floated upward from her earthly body. As she was escorted by the angels, she noticed a spectacular light in the distance. She was being drawn closer and closer to the light. The closer she got, the warmer she felt, until she was totally consumed by this all-loving light. Etta had never known such a feeling of peace and unconditional love than that which she felt coming from the light.

"Welcome, my child. We will now review your life on earth," came a soft, caring voice from the light.

As soon as the voice stopped, Etta saw herself, as if a movie was playing in front of her, but this movie was about her. She stood in the presence of God, and watched as the pictures that flowed in front of her gave an account of her life...

Ancestral History

Lewis Grigsby was born in Greene County, Tennessee, on March 31, 1812. He grew up on a farm and met Rebecca Ann Bryan when he was in his early twenties.

Rebecca was born on April 3, 1818. She was the daughter of Danile (pronounced Dan'l) Bryan, a very prosperous man who held vast land holdings in Del Rio, Tennessee. Rebecca was a very religious woman who attended church regularly. The first church to be built in Del Rio was named Becky's Chapel, in her honor. This building was also used as the first school. Rebecca acquired over 100 acres in land holdings from her father in the Big Creek community of Del Rio.

Lewis and Rebecca married in Greene County, Tennessee, on May 28, 1835. They settled on the land Danile had given to his daughter. There they built a large two-story, wooden-plank house across the road from where the current Del Rio School is located today. The house had a wide front porch which faced the creek that merged with the French Broad River a few miles from their home. They also dug a well which had a hand crank used to draw the water from the well. The remains of the rocks used to build up the wall of the well are still there today.

Lewis and Rebecca were very well-to-do people and were considered to be one of the more prominent families who lived in Del Rio. Lewis was not one who enjoyed physical labor; he had slaves to do the farm work for him. Because of his financial position in the community, he acquired the name of "Colonel Grisby." His favorite pastime was to sit on the front porch and drink whiskey.

The Colonel's behavior totally disgusted Rebecca's father. Danile declared in a voice of rage to his friends, "Well, I know how I'll get rid of 'im! I'll just kill 'im!" Danile brought a 100 gallon barrel of whiskey and set it on the Colonel's front porch. It had a faucet sticking out next to the bottom of the barrel which made the whiskey easily obtainable. Danile was certain that when the Colonel drank all that whiskey it would kill him. The Colonel did drink all of the whiskey and later exclaimed with loud laughter to his friends, as he rubbed his protruding stomach, "He thought he'd kill me, but godsir, he just fattened me!"

Colonel Grigsby and Rebecca had seven children. Their first child, Dan'l (1839-1883) was named after Rebecca's father. He served in the Civil War as a soldier with Company H, First Tennessee Cavalry Division.

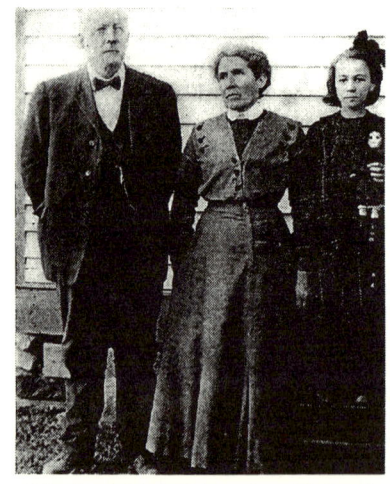

Colonel Lewis Grigsby, Rebecca Bryan Grigsby and daugter, Laura

Their second son was William (1842-1868). John Bryan Grigsby was their third son (1847-1942). His middle name, Bryan, was given to him from his mother's maiden name.

Other children included Thomas (1850-1870); Wiley (1853-?); Joseph C. (1857-?), and their last child was a girl, Laura Grigsby (1859-1941).

Two of Colonel and Rebecca's sons died during the Civil War. They were buried on a plot of ground which was assigned by Colonel Grigsby to be used as the Grigsby Cemetery on what is now Highway 107 in Del Rio. Today it is known as the Stokely Cemetery, probably because Estel Stokely bought the house and land in front of it, and he started burying his relatives there, too.

Colonel Grigsby lived during the administration of 19 different Presidents of the United States, James Madison through Grover Cleveland.

The Colonel was 49 when President Lincoln took office. After the North won the Civil War, he was forced to free his slaves. Some remained on the farm to work because they had no other way of making a living, but they had to be out of Del Rio before dark each day or they risked cruel and inhumane punishment from the whites if caught.

Rebecca Ann Bryan Grigsby died June 20, 1875; Colonel Lewis Grigsby died June 3, 1886.

Third son, John Bryan went by the name of J. B. Grigsby. He was born in 1847 in Del Rio, Tennessee, where he grew up on his parents' farm.

Rebecca managed the money while he was growing up and she saved enough to send him to college in Durham, North Carolina, where he obtained a medical degree at Duke University. He then returned to Del Rio to practice medicine, attending the sick all over the Appalachian Mountains.

J. B. met Rebecca Hurst, and later they were married. They settled on the land J. B. owned in the Meadows Field area of Del Rio. Their house set in a peaceful, open field, which had a small sparkling stream running in front of the house in the distance. J. B. owned the land all the way from where Blue Mill Road and Ground Squirrel Road fork, almost exactly one mile up the road, to Norwood Town Road. He owned the land on both sides of the road that is there today from one mountain to the next. The house that is currently occupied by Doyle and Maude Smith, is where J. B. and Rebecca built their house, about 7/10 of a mile from the fork in the road. The house set on the other side of the creek from the Smiths' house that is there today.

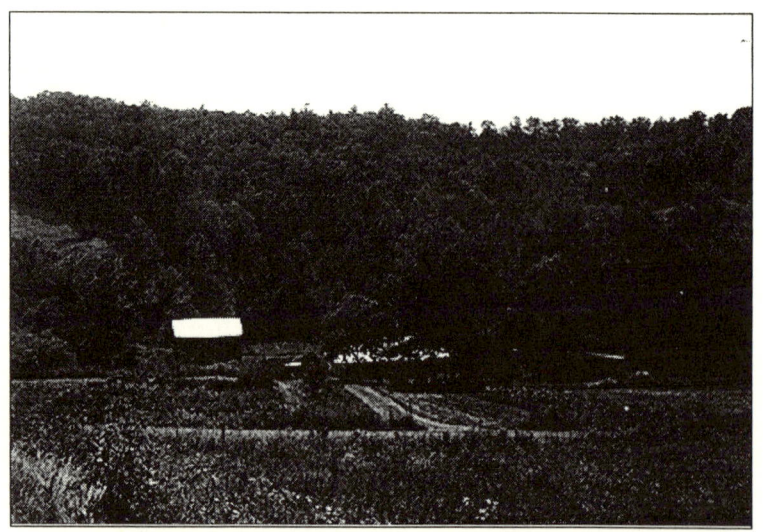

Doyle and Maude Smith currently live on the land that J.B. Grigsby once owned.

J. B. was considered to be gifted at giving names to people and places. He assigned a plot of ground on the mountain in front of the house to be used for a cemetery for the family. He was also the person who assigned the name "London" to the area just before the forks in the road at Blue Mill and Ground Squirrel.

J. B. and Rebecca had four children: Margaret, Henrietta (Sissy), Katie, and John Lewis. The only son, was named after his father and his grandfather. Sissy and Katie both died from tuberculosis, Sissy at age 33, and Katie at age 18.

J. B. divided his land in Meadows Field equally between his only two living children, Margaret and John Lewis. J. B. bought some more land and lived in the house up on the hill that today is remembered as the Tilman Bible home place located in the Nough community (formally called Slabtown). His house set on the hill across the road from the country grocery store known today as Jim Lamb's Grocery.

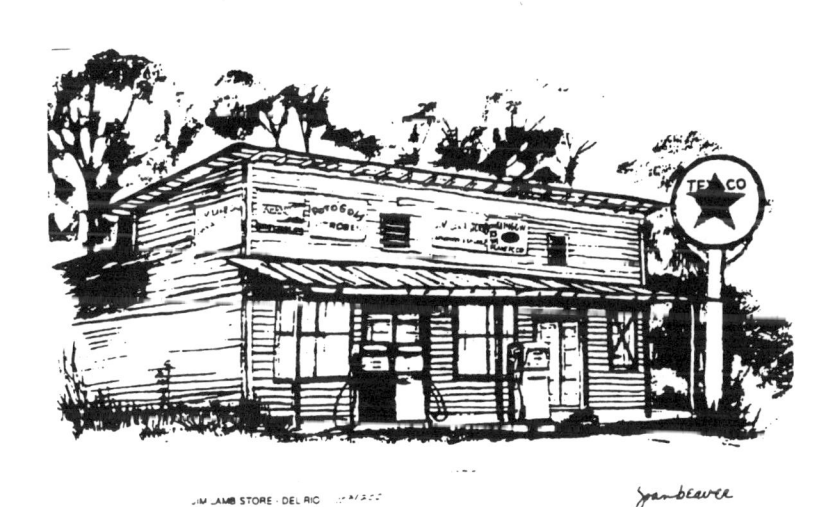

DRAWING BY: JOAN BEAVER

J. B. lived during the Civil War, during which time two of his brothers were killed in the war. He had seen slavery, and he witnessed its abolishment by President Lincoln at the age of seventeen.

Twenty different presidents held office during J. B.'s life: James K. Polk through Calvin Coolidge.

In 1924, J. B. was returning from outside his home late one evening when a shot rang out across the hill where he lived. A bullet from a .22 rifle lodged in his back, killing him at the age of 78. He was buried in the cemetery beside his wife, Rebecca Hurst Grigsby (who had died the previous year on April 8, 1923), on the land he had given to his son, John Lewis.

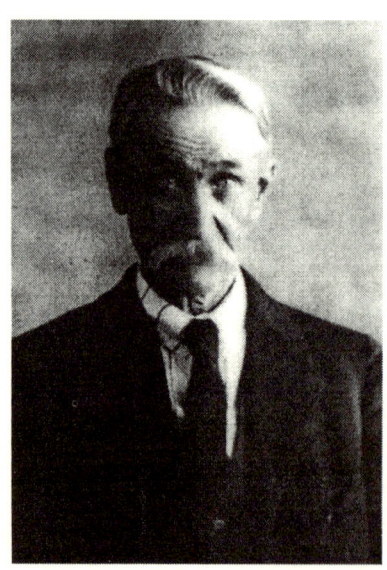

Dr. J. B. Grigsby

John Lewis Grigsby was the fourth and youngest child of J. B. Grigsby and Rebecca Hurst Grigsby. He was born on May 14, 1876, in Del Rio, Tennessee. He was raised on his parents' farm in Meadows Field, where he enjoyed the bounties that came from being a doctor's son.

When he got old enough, John Lewis often went with his father through the mountains on horseback to attend to the sick, or deliver a baby. John Lewis had no formal training as a doctor, but he read his father's medical books and received firsthand training from his father.

When John Lewis was 17, he met Miss Nova Melinda Jane Turner at church. Novie, as she was called by the mountain folks, and her family had moved to Del Rio from North Carolina. Born on June 22, 1877, Novie was the first child of Lige Turner and Nannie Cogdill Turner. She had four siblings: Tom, Carrie, Jessie, and Lisa. Lige was crazy about his little Lisa, but at the tender age of two, she died. Lige became bitter, and he would often abuse his wife and children.

Novie began courting some of the boys of the community, including Lonnie Moore. Lige liked Lonnie and did not want Novie to court anyone else. Novie liked Lonnie, too, but she courted other boys just to spite her father. Novie liked to have a good time. She attended barn dances where she would often stay out all night dancing with Lonnie. She attended corn shuckins' and church socials as often as possible.

When Novie met John Lewis at church, she allowed him to walk her home after the service was over. Lige was sitting in his straight back chair when he saw Novie walking toward the house with John Lewis. He was outraged that she had disobeyed him. When Novie came through the door, her father sprang from his chair and asked her in his high-tempered voice, "What did you let John Lewis Grigsby walk you home fer?!" Lige kept a hog rifle over the mantel above the fireplace to ward off any predators that came around the house. He reached up over the mantel and took down the gun. "Well, I'll jest kill ye! I'll jest kill ye and end it all!" said Lige in a ferocious tone. He was insane with anger towards Novie, and she knew he would kill her, but just as he turned the gun toward her, Nannie, Novie's mother, screamed from where she stood in the front doorway diverting Lige's attention to her.

"Oh Lord! I see Lisa a'comin'! I see Lisa a'comin'!" shouted Nannie hysterically as she gazed up at the evening sky.

Lige's attention was drawn away from Novie as he slowly put the gun down. He was astonished at his wife's outburst.

Had Lisa's spirit really come back to save her older sister, or was this just a clever maneuver from Nannie to stop her husband from killing their first born? Novie never knew the answer, but she was convinced it had saved her life.

Novie was desperate to get away from her overbearing father. She would sneak around to see John Lewis behind her father's back. On June 23, 1894, John Lewis and Novie snuck away and visited E. B. Crowder, M. G., where he united the two in the holy bonds of matrimony. John Lewis was eighteen years old, and Novie was seventeen years old.

John Lewis Grigsby and Nova Melinda Jane Turner Grigsby were just one couple out of many who experienced hard mountain times. They had only been married about four months when Novie became pregnant with their first child. In August, 1895, John and Novie had a son. They named him Lewis, his father's middle name. They were very proud of their first born.

John Lewis raised tobacco and farmed to provide for his family, a lifestyle very different from the comfortable life he experienced while growing up as the son of a doctor. Novie tended to their son and managed the household chores. On May 19, 1897, Novie gave birth to another baby. This time it was a little redheaded girl. They named her Carrie Etta Grigsby.

List Of Articles and Interviews Etta Nichols Appeared In*

1976 October	The Newport Plain Talk—60th Wedding Anniversary
1979 March	*Redneck Mothers. Good Ol' Girls, and Other Southern Belles*—Book
1981 March	The Knoxville News-Sentinel—Personal Interview
1981 August	The Newport Plain Talk—Personal Interview
1982 May	The Newport Plain Talk—Baby born on Etta's Birthday
1983 October 11	The Knoxville Journal—Hamilton's Baby Story
1983 October 19	The Knoxville Journal Newspaper—Personal Interview
1984	The Associated Press—Personal Interview
1984	The Knoxville Journal—Personal Interview
1984 February	AARP Magazine—Photo and Short Article

1984 Summer	The Heartland Series—Episode XXV—"Midwife"
1984 December	Tennessee Cooperator Magazine—She's A Living Legend
1985	STAR Magazine—Personal Interview
1985 September	The Atlanta Journal and Constitution—Legend As Midwife of the Mtns.
1985 October 11	NBC Nightly News with Tom Brokaw—National News Interview
1985 October	The Newport Plain Talk—NBC News Staff at Etta's Article
1986 January	Tennessee Homecoming Calendar—Appears on the Month of January
1986 January	The Newport Plain Talk—Winner of Calendar Contest
1986 March	The Newport Plain Talk—Most Notable Resident
1986 April	The Newport Plain Talk—Our View Point
1986 April	People
1986 May	NATIONAL GEOGRAPHIC, Vol. 169, No. 5
1986 October	The Newport Plain Talk—Sutton Family From Nashville
1986 November	The Greeneville Sun—Personal Interview

1987 May	The Newport Plain Talk—90th Birthday
1987 June 12	The Newport Plain Talk—Agency to Honor Midwife
1987 June	The Newport Plain Talk—Humanitarian Award Winner
1987 July 24	The Newport Plain Talk—Delivers Twins at Age Ninety
1988 May	The Newport Plain Talk—Celebrates Ninety-First Birthday
1994 November	The Citizen Tribune—Article on Etta's Death
1994 November	The Newport Plain Talk—Article on Etta's Death
*Author's note:	There may be more articles about Etta Nichols, but these are all I uncovered during my research.

PART I

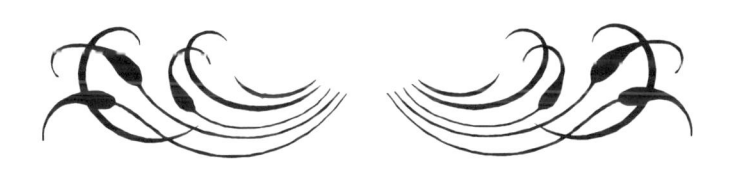

Life Growing Up

PART I

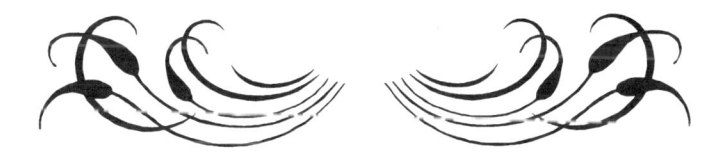

Life Growing Up

Carrie Etta Grigsby was born in an area called Meadows Field, in Del Rio, Tennessee, on May 19, 1897. Later her parents, John Lewis Grigsby and Novie Grigsby, added Margaret to her name, after John's sister. Her name became Margaret Carrie Etta Grigsby, although Margaret was not added to the birth certificate.

Etta lived in a little red cabin her father built on some land that his father, J. B. Grigsby, had deeded to him, along with her parents, and her older brother, Lewis.

Etter, as the mountain people called her, was a happy child who was known to laugh a lot as she was growing up. She had pretty red hair that hung in curls, and a rosy complexion which complemented her sparkling blue eyes. Her dress, made of white cotton, came down to her petite ankles and possessed long puffy sleeves which stopped just below her elbow. She wore thick white cotton stockings which covered her entire legs from her ankles to the top of her thighs. Her shoes were made of leather with a tiny strap crossing over the top of her foot to a fastener on the side, although from May through October the children did not wear shoes. It was seen as a waste by Etta's mother and most other mountain people to wear shoes in the warm months of the year.

On August 31, 1899, Novie gave birth to her third child, a son named Waitsel. Etta was two years old; Lewis was four.

The Grigsby family was growing, and life became harder with each passing day for John Lewis and Novie. Three weeks after Waitsel was born, tragedy struck their happy family. Little Lewis had been sick with membranous croup, as it was called. Lewis started coughing. Novie and John noticed something was wrong. Lewis was choking on phlegm! Etta watched helplessly as her frightened parents worked frantically with their firstborn, trying desperately to dislodge the mucus from Lewis' airway, but they were unsuccessful. Lewis died at the tender age of four. He was buried in the cemetery on the mountain in front of John and Novie's house which J. B. had assigned to be used as the family cemetery when he first moved there.

Months passed. Etta was now three years old, and her mother was pregnant with her fourth child. Life was a struggle for John Lewis, trying to keep his family fed and clothed. Some people left the harshness of the mountains behind and moved to places where, hopefully, life would be kinder.

John's sister, Margaret, and her husband, Mack Bailey, sold the land J. B. deeded to her in order to get the money to move to Washington State. The thought of joining her was more tempting to John Lewis every day, but he could not go while Novie was pregnant. It would be too much for a "woman with child" to withstand. He would have to endure the mountain's hardships for a while longer.

When she was four, Etta had another brother enter the world. He was named Paul. He was born in 1901.

Chores were assigned to the children at a very young age. Etta helped her mother in the kitchen by washing the dishes after every meal. Being only four years old, she could not reach the dishpan on the kitchen table; she had to put the dishpan in the seat of a straightback chair in order to carry out her assigned chore. She carefully removed the dishes from the table and placed them in the dishpan. She always turned her plates up and stacked the glasses in around them. One night she put the dishes in hot water which had been heated on the wood cook stove. She put her hands in the hot water and quickly jerked them back out; the water was too hot! She walked over to the tin bucket which contained the family's drinking water and dipped out some cold water with the long-handled water dipper, then poured it into the dishpan. Every dish and glass in the dishpan cracked into multiple pieces. Etta stood looking at the broken dishes in disbelief. "What kind of punishment will I get fer doin' this?" Etta wondered to herself. Etta left the dishes in the dishpan and did not say anything to her mother about the incident as she quietly got ready for bed. She wanted to put off her punishment for as long as possible. The next morning Novie went into the kitchen only to find she had no plates or glasses. Novie knew Etta would not break the dishes on purpose, so she never punished her. Etta exclaimed to Waitsel in a sigh of relief, "I just knowed I wuz gonna' get a whoppin' fer doin' that!" Of course Waitsel was too young to care, but he was the only person she could confide in that was close to her own age.

Novie was very strict with her children. She had been raised to believe in many of the old-timey ways of how to teach a child a certain lesson when the child made a mistake. One morning four-year-old Etta accidentally wet the bed. She walked into the kitchen where Novie was preparing breakfast and said in a sorrowful tone, "Mommie, I peed in the bed, and my clothes are wet."

Novie walked over and grabbed Etta by the back of her little cotton gown, and pushed her into the bedroom. She took hold of Etta by the back of the head, and shoved her face down into the soaked sheets. "Now, let this be a lesson to you, young lady! Don't you ever do that agin, or you'll get more of this next time. Do you hear me?!" Novie shouted in a frightening tone.

Poor little Etta looked up at her mother apprehensively, "No, Mommie. I promise I won't."

"Now get yourself in some dry clothes, and take those wet sheets off the bed," Novie ordered.

Etta did as her mother told her as the tears streamed down her rose-colored cheeks. She had to be careful not to let her mother hear her whimpers, or she feared she would be punished again. Once Etta had followed her mother's instructions, she went into the kitchen to eat her breakfast. She was silent at the table as she ate her eggs, gravy, and biscuits. Once finished, she cleared the dishes from the table and began her chores.

Etta had trouble sleeping for several nights after her horrible experience. She was afraid she might wet the bed again if she fell asleep, and she certainly did not want to go through that appalling punishment again. Her fear was seated deep within her subconscious, which awakened her before she had any future "accidents." When Etta realized she could control her "urges to go" she began sleeping peacefully throughout the night once more.

Two years passed. John and Novie had put moving to Washington out of their minds, for the time being, anyway. Novie had been "with child" once more, her fifth pregnancy, but had miscarried. A few months later she became pregnant again. Etta was six years old: Waitsel was four; Paul was two.

Summer arrived after a cool spring brought new beauty to the mountains. It was time to do some spring cleaning inside the house. John Lewis took the stove pipes down from their wood cook stove in the kitchen and poured the soot into a large bucket. He placed the bucket on the floor in the front room as he walked outside with the stovepipes under his arms. He went to the creek to wash the pipes off. Novie was outside talking to a neighbor. While Etta and Waitsel were left unsupervised in the front room, they found the temptation to play in the soot too hard to resist. Etta walked over to the bucket and stuck her hand down into the soot. It felt soft and silky.

She liked the way it felt on her skin. She lowered her arm down even further until the soot was up to her elbow. Suddenly Etta jerked her hand out of the bucket with a handful of soot and threw it all over Waitsel. Waitsel joined Etta at the bucket. Soon the children were covered from head to toe with the black soot. There was soot all over the floor, on the furniture, and on the walls! The children were having a great time...until their mother walked in.

"Lordy, mercy! What'er you kids a'doin?!" Novie yelled as she entered the door.

All that could be seen of the children were the whites of their eyes as they were opened wide in surprise at having been caught in the act of their mischief. Etta and Waitsel were silent and still as they stood awaiting their fate. They both received a "good thrashin'" from Novie. This was one lesson Etta nor Waitsel would ever forget.

Novie enjoyed dipping snuff. She noticed Etta staring at her one afternoon as if she wished she could have some. Novie looked back at Etta for a moment then told her, "Etter, go out back and get me n' you a brush, and I'll give you a snoot of snuff."

"Oh, Mommie, you won't," answered Etta, thinking her mother was only teasing her.

"Oh, yes I will," replied Novie in a tone of certitude.

Etta was excited to the core as she ran hurriedly out the back door to a nearby birch tree. People used the birch twigs to make toothbrushes. They broke off the size they wanted, then beat the end until it became soft and prickly. Etta broke a twig off for her mother then she broke off a larger one for herself. She beat the ends of the twigs with a rock until they were soft, then she ran back inside to her mother in the front room.

Novie asked Etta, "Why did you get such a big brush for yourself?"

"Cause I want a big ol' dip of that!" answered Etta enthusiastically.

"Okay, put the brush inside your mouth and get it good n' wet."

Etta did as her mother instructed.

"Now let me have it an' I'll swab you some snuff on it," said Novie.

"Mommie, let me get it," begged Etta.

"Why no. I'll get it fer ye," answered Novie.

"No, you won't get me enough," whined Etta.

Novie took the brush and started rolling it over in the snuff.

"Get it real good n' full, Mommie."

Novie handed the brush back to Etta. She stood there looking at the snuff, as if she were in a daze. She was afraid it would burn her after she got it.

"Put it in your mouth," challenged Novie.

Etta put the snuff in her mouth and just about the time it got wet, Novie said, "Swoller it!"

Etta could tell by her mother's tone of voice that she was serious. She swallowed the snuff and immediately her throat felt as if every bit of the hide had been taken off. She ran into the kitchen to get a dipper full of water. There was not a drop of water in the bucket! The coffee pot with cold coffee left from the morning's breakfast was still on the stove. Etta grabbed it and frantically drank every drop of coffee in it. Etta was furious that her mother had done that to her. She believed her mother had poured the drinking water out while she was outside getting their brushes. Novie came and stood in the doorway going into the kitchen. Etta set the coffee pot down and walked outside. She stayed gone for a long time. Etta overheard her mother telling her father later, "I had to make her sick on it. I couldn't dip with no satisfaction knowin' she wuz wantin' a dip." That was the one and only time Etta ever had the urge to try dipping snuff.

On February 17, 1904, Novie gave birth to her fifth child. She was a cuddly little redheaded baby girl. They named her Alverta, but the mountain folks called her Alvertie. Etta was delighted to finally get a sister. They would grow up to be very dear to one another.

Paul, the third and youngest son of John Lewis and Novie, was scooting Etta's little chair over the kitchen floor while he was playing one day. The chair was made just the right size for a child. Oh, he was having a ball pretending he was guiding a team of horses. He went into the "meal room," a special small room used to store barrels of meal and flour. Paul opened each barrel and peeped inside. He looked up and said to his mother, who was cooking supper just outside the room, "Daddy's a good'un, ain't he? The meal barrel and the flour barrel is nearly full!" Paul was a very bright youngster.

When Paul was four, he developed a bad case of whooping cough, which matured into a fatal case of tuberculosis. He was buried in the family cemetery beside his brother, Lewis, who had also died at the age of four.

A few months later John Lewis made a trip, along with his Uncle Wiley, to Molson, Washington. Uncle Wiley

Etta "Granny" Nichols—Last of the Old-Timey Midwives

owned some land and a small cabin there. John Lewis left his family in Meadows Field until he earned enough money to buy them train tickets to move out there with him. John drove a stagecoach until the money was raised.

Upon John Lewis' return to Del Rio, he bought a big doll for Etta, who had been fighting a bout of pneumonia fever. She became very excited when her daddy gave her the doll. She had never seen such a big doll; it was almost as big as she was. She would cherish this doll for as long as she lived.

Once Etta recovered from her illness, the family packed up their belongings and waited to board the train at the Del Rio Depot. Etta was eight years old, Waitsel was six, and Alvertie was almost two.

Etta was so excited to get to ride on a train; she had never been on one before now. Novie sat with the children inside the depot as they waited for the train to pull in, while John Lewis made pleasant conversation with some

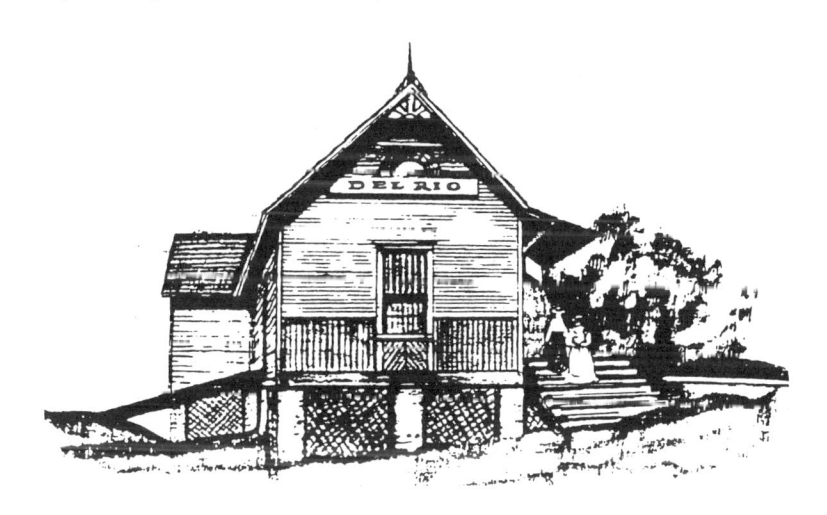

DEL RIO'S FIRST DEPOT
DRAWING BY: JOAN BEAVER

of the local men who spent much of their day hanging around the depot passing the time. Etta jumped up from her seat when she heard the train coming down the tracks. The steam engine left a trail of smoke behind as it came around the bend toward the depot. The Grigsby family walked down the wide wooden steps at the depot's entrance to board the train, while a railroad employee wheeled their belongings to the baggage car off the ramp on the other side of the building.

The train ride seemed endless for Novie, who was having a hard time keeping Alvertie occupied. The train conductor tried his best to get Novie to give Alvertie to him. She was the cutest child he had ever seen. He was immediately stricken with love for this little girl. Novie was afraid he might try to steal her, so she had to keep a very close eye on her.

Etta was spellbound as she gazed at all the new sights from her window. The further away from Tennessee they traveled, the flatter the land became. Etta had never been able to see for such a long distance across the country as she could see now. All the scenery was so different from what she was used to, and she loved to hear the whistle coming from the engine as they neared a town. What an adventure for an eight-year-old girl who had never been out of Del Rio.

When the long train ride finally ended, Uncle Wiley met them at the train depot in Molson with his wagon and team of horses to take them to his cabin. The Grigsby family now had a new home in a place much different from the one they left behind. Uncle Wiley's cabin consisted of two rooms. One had two beds with an oil lamp on a small handmade wooden table between them. The other room was a kitchen only large enough to hold a wood stove, a small eating table, and a cupboard for dishes and other kitchen supplies. Another oil lamp was on the kitchen table.

Days passed. After supper, Etta cleared the dirty dishes from the table and washed them by the light of the oil lamp, which bestowed a flickering illumination on the bare walls. When she was finished, she and the other children brushed their teeth with beaten birch twigs and soda. After a hard day of playing and helping with her brother and sister, Etta was ready to settle down in her pallet she made each night on the floor. Alvertie slept with John and Novie, while Waitsel shared a bed with Uncle Wiley.

John and Novie raised vegetables, wheat, oats, barley, rye, and milked 11 cows to earn their living. The work started with the first cock's crow at dawn and did not end until well past dusk, when the men came in from the fields. The milking was done by the children and Novie.

Etta and Waitsel attended the school in Molson, about a mile away from the cabin. They walked to and from school each day. One of the girls at school started going around singing a song mockingly, while skipping around Etta.

"Redhead, gingerbread, five cents a loaf," the girl squealed in the tune of Red Rover, Red Rover. She sang this repeatedly each day.

Etta got agitated after several days of this. She had lost all her patience with the girl. The next time the girl started singing she grabbed the girl by the arm and warned her in a harsh tone, "Don't you call me that no more, unless you want a good thrashin'!" The little girl never bothered Etta or spoke of her red hair again.

Etta was frightened one day by an Indian who rode by on his horse while she was outside the cabin playing. He stopped, some distance away, and sat on his horse looking long and closely at her. He did this several times. The children at school teased Etta that the Indian wanted her scalp. They could have been right, because she had beautiful long, red hair that lay in curls all down her back. The Indian stopped coming after awhile. Maybe he realized he was scaring her.

Novie became "with child" once more after the move to Washington. She was riding a horse one day when it bolted and jumped the corral fence, causing Novie to miscarry. John took the baby and buried it under a big cypress tree in the distance from the house. He marked the grave with a rock that gave the appearance of an eagle with its wings outstretched.

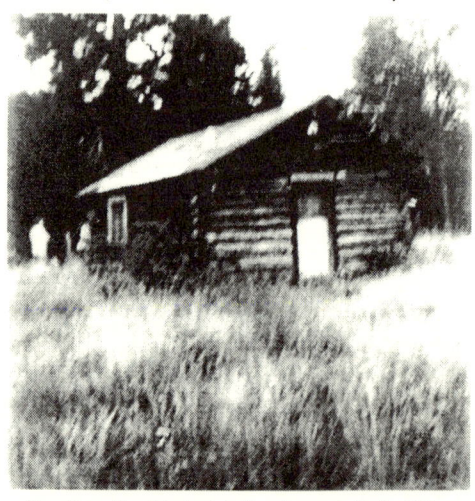

One of the cabins John Lewis built, as it appeared in the 1970s

After three years, John Lewis and Novie were both homesick for Del Rio. They decided after some discussion the time had come to move back home. They packed their belongings and boarded the train back to Tennessee. When the Grigsby family returned to Del Rio in 1908, they settled back into their previous home at Meadows Field.

Etta was now 11 years old. She was responsible for looking after her younger siblings, and doing the chores around the house, such as sweeping, washing dishes, fluffing the feather tick mattresses, and straightening the covers. She also helped with the milking each morning and night because Novie was now pregnant with another child.

On July 13, 1909, Novie gave birth to another baby girl. They named her Emily Willie Grigsby. She had a fair complexion and lighter hair than Etta's and Alvertie's. She was the sixth child of John Lewis and Novie. Later in life Emily Willie took the nickname of "Bill."

John Lewis had learned about treating the sick from going with his father, J. B., and also by reading his medical books. Many were the times the mountain folk would ride on horseback to J B.'s house in need of a doctor, only to find him gone on another case. J. B. was the only medi-

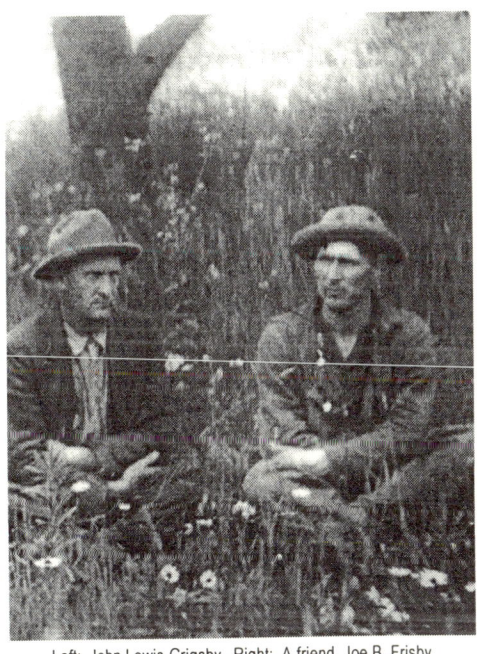

Left: John Lewis Grigsby. Right: A friend, Joe B. Frisby

cal doctor the people of the mountains had, unless they made the journey to Newport, some 20 miles away.

John Lewis was awakened one night by a loud knock on his door. He got up to see who it was. As he opened the door he was almost run over by a hysterical man. "Please, will ye come with me? My wife is ready to give birth, n' Doc ain't at home!" the man said in a panic. John Lewis went with the man, delivered the baby, and was paid with two laying hens.

It did not take long for word to spread about John Lewis' knowledge of medicine. People started coming to him as often as they did his father. It seemed to him that babies always wanted to enter the world in the wee hours of the morning. He was awakened many times after midnight by the frantic banging on his door. "I'm afraid my wife will have the baby before we get there," a nervous father would say.

John would answer, "Well, go saddle up my mare while I get my clothes on." The men would ride on the trails through the dark mountains until they reached their destination. There was always a midwife present to assist the "doctor" during childbirth.

Etta had always been interested in becoming a nurse as she was growing up. She asked her father, "Daddy, can I go with you next time you go out doctorin'?"

"No!" came the quick reply from her mother.

"Why, let'er go, Novie. If she wants to learn doctorin' leave 'er alone an' let 'er learn it," said John Lewis.

Etta was almost 13 and started going with her father every chance she could. She became very helpful during deliveries. She learned about medicine from watching her father, just as he had learned from watching his father.

John Lewis had his own "little black bag" in which he kept powdered medicine wrapped up in little papers. He had a set of scales which allowed him to weigh the medicine according to law by milligram, grain, etc. He would take the bottle of medicine he ordered from Eli Lilly & Park Davis Company, and measure out a two-month supply of single doses into the paper containers. They were deposited into his medical bag along with a bottle of ether, clean rags, and his own home remedies which he made from mountain herbs. Spikenard was one of his favorites to give to people who had nothing seriously wrong; they just felt "poorly." Spikenard belongs to the ginseng family and has an aromatic root. John Lewis would beat the roots into a powder then boil it in water to make a kind of tea for his patient to drink. He would use beeswood leaves boiled in water as a drink that helped with kidney problems. To treat "the itch," polk root was boiled in water then the solution was spread over the skin. Head lice were killed with the root from the larkspur flower, a genus of plants of the buttercup family. The root was boiled, then the solution was poured over the head.

Most of the people living in the mountains believed in planting their gardens and their crops by the signs of the moon; John Lewis was no exception. He had seen corn grow 20 feet tall with skinny stalks and small ears of corn from not planting it during the correct sign. If it was planted during the appropriate sign of the moon, the cornstalk would be short and bear big, delicious ears of corn.

There were also "moon babies." According to the mountain people, if a child was born during the wrong sign of the moon he would be unruly, getting into all kinds of mischief as he grew up. They also believed that a "woman with child" should cover herself from head to toe, if having her picture made. To show one's face in a photograph while pregnant would surely bring bad luck to the mother and the baby.

Another mountain superstition involved taking baths. Some of the people believed that if a person sat in a tub of water too long their body would "suck up" the water through their bowels and they would explode. Needless to say, these people did not spend much time in the wash tub come Saturday, the day considered to be bath day.

Etta continued to go with her father on "baby cases" throughout the mountains. She had the equivalent of an eighth-grade education, although she only went to school for three years while living in Molson, Washington. When she was going to school, children of all ages sat together in one room, learning how to read, write, and do arithmetic. Some history and geography were also taught. Once students learned all of the information in their school books, they were considered to be graduated from the eighth grade. Etta wanted desperately to go to nurse's school, but her father could not afford to send her, and Novie needed her to help with the household chores and watch after the children.

When Etta was 13 her father decided to move back to Molson, Washington. John Lewis traveled alone by train once more. He stayed with his sister, Margaret, and her husband, Mack Bailey, this time until he was able to build a cabin for his growing family.

John took up a land grant for 40 acres next to where his Uncle Wiley lived. After the rest of the family arrived in Washington, they settled into their new home and the daily routine of chores. This time John raised cattle and sheep to support his family while Novie sewed all the children's clothes, and made butter and buttermilk. She also made lye soap from hog fat left over in the fall after the hogs were slaughtered. Clothes were washed on a washboard using the lye soap, then put into a large kettle of boiling water. Using a big stick, Etta would stand over the pot and stir the clothes to sterilize them. The clothes were then put through a wringer before hanging them out on the clothesline to dry. A small iron, made of cast iron was set over the fire until heated, then used to iron the wrinkles out of the clothes.

The children played in the creek through the week to help rid themselves of some of the soil and sweat their bodies accumulated from one Saturday to the next. When Saturday arrived a big round washtub was filled with heated water from the wood stove in the kitchen. One by one the children would all take their "Saturday bath" in order to be nice and clean for Sunday's church services.

One evening Etta was outside hanging laundry when she noticed something jumping over the corral fence. She was terrified at first, because she thought it was a huge rabbit. She had always heard the rabbits got big in this part of the country, but this rabbit was as big as a kangaroo! The animal hopped towards Mr. Marshall's place, a nearby neighbor. Etta went running to her father in the cornfield. "Daddy, there wuz a huge wild animal just hopped over our fence and headed fer the Marshalls'!" Etta said excitedly as she tried to get her breath. John Lewis got on his horse and headed in the direction Etta pointed. Later that evening he returned with a deer mounted across his horse. Etta laughed at herself for mistaking a deer for a big rabbit. The family enjoyed eating deer meat for many weeks to follow.

Novie had given birth to another son not long after arriving in Molson. They named him Creed. He was almost a year and a half old now, but he was not learning as quickly as the other children did. It became quite obvious Creed was mentally handicapped. Someone had to keep an eye on him at all times.

The Grigsby family spent almost two years in Washington when, once again, they became homesick for Tennessee. John Lewis sold his 40 acres of land to his Uncle Wiley for $40 so he would have the money to buy the train tickets for his family to move back home. When they arrived in Del Rio they settled back into their home at Meadows Field once more.

John Lewis decided he could be a financial success if he just had enough money to build a sawmill. He went to George Runnion and gave him a deed of trust on his land in order to get the money to build the sawmill. He built it on the other side of the creek from where their house stood. A water flume created an inclined channel for directing the water which ran from Blue Mill all the way down below Slabtown. The flume ran close to the creek behind John Lewis' sawmill. When the slabs of wood reached a particular section of the community they spilled over and fell into the road. Slabs of wood lay all over the ground and in the road; thus the name "Slabtown" was adopted for this small area of the community. Some of the people in the community resented the name given to their neighborhood, so it was later named Nough, for Charles Goodnough, a resident, but the name of "Slabtown" would be carried down through many future generations to come for this area.

The winters were harsh and bitterly cold in the Appalachian Mountains. The children had to walk four miles to attend school at Mulberry Gap. Their feet and legs would be numb from wading through the snow. But, being children, they made each day fun by playing in the light, fluffy, white stuff. Snowballs came whirling from behind the trees, hitting an unsuspecting student in the face as he approached the school. The children could hardly wait until recess came so they could go out and play in the snow and pay back their hidden attackers who had struck on the way to school. Snowball fights were a favorite game of all the children at school in the wintertime. When they arrived home in the afternoon they warmed themselves by the woodstove. Etta usually fixed them a treat of creamy, cold snowcream after their chores were completed. They loved her snowcream, and Etta liked it, too.

On November 16, 1912, John Lewis' and Novie's eighth child made his appearance into the world. He was their fifth son. They named him Lurlie.

It was hog-killing season again. John Lewis and Waitsel killed several hogs each year to help put food on the table. The hog meat fed the family all winter long, along with vegetables Etta and Novie canned from the summer garden. Sausage and livermush were also made from the hog meat. Etta added just the right amount of spices to make the whole family's mouths water in anticipation.

The years passed by quickly, bringing with them another son for John Lewis and Novie, born on March 16, 1915. They named him Furman.

Etta walked four miles with her family to church at Mulberry Gap each Sunday. She was 18 now, and had her eye on a young man by the name of James Harrison Nichols, whom she met at church. Etta had not been seriously interested in courting any man until she met Harrison. She had been kept busy helping her mother at home. Harrison started walking Etta home from church after each service. They went on hayrides and attended social gatherings together. They courted for a little over one year before Harrison swallowed the lump in his throat and proposed marriage to Etta. Etta discussed Harrison's proposal with her parents before giving him an answer. The next time she saw Harrison she agreed to become his wife.

On October 15, 1916, Harrison and Etta went to the home of Ishom Stinson, who lived a mile or so away in Bear Holler. There they were married by Jimmy M. Jones, Esq. Ishom Stinson and Claude Nichols, Harrison's only full brother, were the witnesses. Harrison and Etta were now ready to embark upon their new life together as husband and wife.

PART II

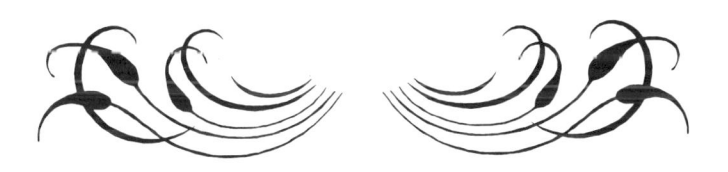

Married Life

PART II

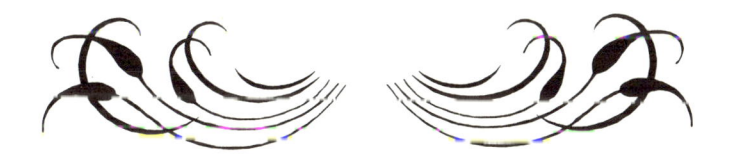

Married Life

Harrison Nichols was the first son of Millard Nichols and Martha Cordelia Clements Nichols. He was born October 14, 1896. He had one younger full brother, Claude Nichols. Harrison's father died from "the fever" when Harrison was just a young boy. His mother, Martha, remarried after several years and gave birth to twin boys, Clayton and Clyde Crowder. Martha had a twin, too, named Mary. After the birth of the twin boys came Thora, Lula, Roy, and Pearl Crowder. The children grew up on a small farm in Del Rio in an area known as Bear Branch.

After they were first married, Harrison and Etta lived with John Lewis and Novie. Etta became pregnant soon after. Novie discovered she, too, was pregnant a few weeks after Etta made her announcement.

Harrison helped in the fields and the sawmill while Etta continued her household chores. John Lewis added more rooms to their small house after acquiring the sawmill. It was now spacious enough for all the family to live comfortably. The downstairs contained a large kitchen, and a front room had two beds, several straightback chairs, and a fireplace. There were two bedrooms downstairs, while the upstairs contained several more straw-tick mattresses where the boys slept. There were no walls; it was just one large open space upstairs. The floors were made from yellow poplar, which were scrubbed clean with Red Devil lye soap.

The time came to send for a midwife for Etta. Mary Bible Smith had delivered numerous babies. Harrison journeyed on horseback to retrieve her from her home across from Walnut Holler, up the road several miles from Midway.

It had been two days since Mary arrived to help deliver Etta's baby; it still had not come. "The first child always takes its time. Ain't no need to try an' rush it. It'll git here when it's good n' ready," John Lewis told Etta.

Novie was not too far from being ready to have her baby, and with Etta in the bed, no one was cooking. Mary was getting hungrier by the minute. Novie's brother, Tom Turner, and his wife lived up the road from John Lewis and Novie. Mrs. Turner came to visit on Mary's second day there. She could tell Mary was hungry. She returned on the third day with a big plate of greens she picked from the woods, new potatoes, cornbread, and a big glass of buttermilk. Mary ate as if she were about to starve to death. Mary's voice was filled with gratitude as she told Mrs. Turner, "That's the best dinner I've eat in all my life!"

Harrison was out in the field working when Mary sent Alvertie out to fetch him. The time had come. John Lewis was gone; he would miss the opportunity of delivering his first grandchild. Harrison came running to the house when Alvertie told him the time had come. He pulled up a chair on the front porch and sat down. He leaned the back of the chair against the wall as he waited anxiously for his firstborn to arrive. Mary and Novie tried several times to get Harrison to come inside and help since John Lewis was not there. They wanted Harrison to stand over Etta and let her pull on his arm when she had a bearing-down pain; it would help her to be able to push harder. Novie could not help Etta since she was ready to deliver soon herself. On their last attempt to get Harrison to help he just looked down at his feet, shook his head, and replied, "No taters! No taters!" He was not about to enter a room where a woman was giving birth. Novie got so angry with Harrison she raked him over the coals for not being willing to help his wife. Etta gave one strong push and a red, wrinkled little baby girl entered the world. Mary tied the umbilical cord then cut it. She held the baby upside down by her feet and smacked her little bottom. Hearing a loud cry, Harrison realized he was now a father. Mary cleaned the baby up and put her in a soft baby gown and blanket. She placed her in Etta's arms then went outside to tell Harrison he had a daughter. It was July 30, 1917, when Harrison and Etta became the proud parents of Emily Laura Nichols.

Three weeks after Etta gave birth to her first child Novie gave birth to another son on August 17, 1917. He was named after his father, except his middle name was spelled differently. John Louis Grigsby became the newest member of the Grigsby family. To avoid confusion, they would call him J. L.

John Lewis had not been as successful in the lumber business as he had hoped. As a matter of fact, it looked as if he was going to lose his land to George Runnion. John Lewis could not let that happen. He went to the courthouse in Newport and put all his land in Waitsel's name. Somehow John Lewis knew he would find a way to pay Mr. Runnion the money he had borrowed from him.

Novie often sat on the front porch talking to female visitors, leaving Alvertie in charge of watching Creed, who was six years old now. On this particular day, Novie had been outside for hours. Alvertie was growing tired from having to keep a constant eye on her little brother. They were in the front room of the house. There was a straightback chair in front of the fireplace with the back turned towards the fire. A garment was draped over the back of the chair to dry.

Alvertie was on the other side of the room from the fireplace. Creed made a run for the chair and climbed up on it. Before Alvertie could get to him, Creed started climbing up the back of the chair. It toppled over, throwing Creed into the fireplace. Alvertie screamed for her mother as she tried to drag Creed from the burning em-

Etta "Granny" Nichols—Last of the Old-Timey Midwives

bers. Novie rushed inside to see what had happened. In a panic Novie yelled for John Lewis who was working down at the sawmill. John Lewis came running up to the house when he heard the terror in Novie's cries. Creed had been severely burned over most of his upper body. John Lewis sent for his father, J. B. While awaiting his father's arrival John Lewis peeled the scorched clothing from his son's burnt body as the boy lay on the bed in torturous pain. J. B. came quickly to aid his grandson. He first cleaned the burnt areas, then he rubbed the burns with a special healing salve before wrapping clean, white clothes loosely around the burned areas of Creed's body. J. B. gave his grandson what he could for the pain, but he was not very hopeful that Creed would make it, although he did not tell John Lewis or Novie of his doubts. A couple of days passed. Pneumonia set in on little Creed's lungs, caused from the burns to his chest. He died at the age of six. He was buried in the family cemetery beside his two older brothers, Lewis and Paul.

Several months later Harrison and Etta decided to move to Virginia. Harrison knew he could make more money working in the coal mines than he could as a farmer. They made the arrangements for their move, packed up what little they owned, and boarded the train in Del Rio to begin their journey to Tom Creek, Virginia. Upon their arrival Harrison and Etta found a small house close to town where most of the other mining families lived. They settled into their house and began their new life together with the same hopes and dreams all young married couples have—to provide a good home for their children with plenty of food to eat and the love of God in their heart.

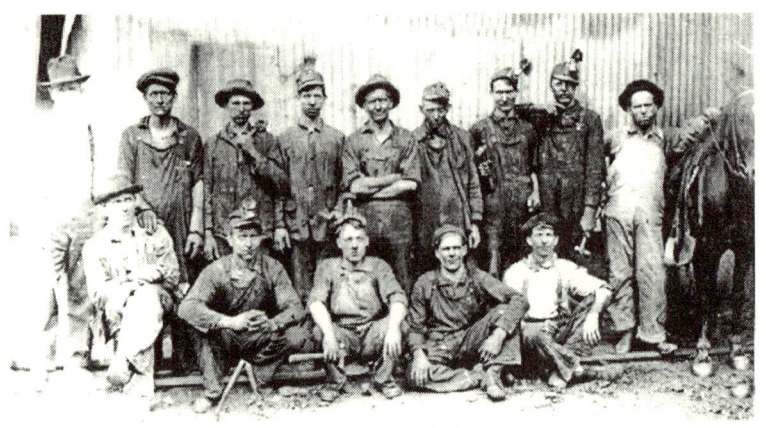

Harrison Nichols stands third from left

Harrison and Etta lived in Virginia for over a year. Mining was hard, backbreaking work and very dangerous. Etta feared the news would come each day that Harrison had been trapped in a cave-in at the mines. She was also homesick for her family in Del Rio because she was now pregnant with her second child and needed her mother's help with Emily on days she was too sick to tend to her properly. Harrison knew they would have to leave before Etta became any "bigger with child," or she would not be able to make the journey. Harrison collected his wages at the end of the week and informed his boss he would not be back; he was moving his family back to Tennessee. When Harrison arrived home Etta had their belongings packed. The journey home began.

In Del Rio, Harrison took Etta and Emily to Novie's, where they were greeted with loving affection from all the family members. Etta was so happy to be back home! She had always had a close bond with her family, and she had missed them terribly during her stay in Virginia. A few days later Harrison learned of a farmhouse for rent

Etta "Granny" Nichols—Last of the Old-Timey Midwives

on the Nathan Huff estate in the area known as The Fifteenth. Harrison and Etta moved into the house and Harrison became a sharecropper while Etta tended to Emily and the household chores.

Etta became acquainted with Flora Corn and her 11-year-old daughter, Opal, who lived up The Fifteenth road close to the mission school in Morgan's Gap after she and Harrison moved to the Huff farm.

Flora and Opal were visiting Etta one day when Opal started telling Etta about a young woman named Leonora Whitaker who had come to the Mission in 1912 at the age of 19 to help teach the mountain children in school.

"She come all the way from Asheville, North Carolina, just a girl herself, to these untamed mountains to help us!" Opal exclaimed in her girlish excitement. "I want to be a teacher, too. Hearing my mother tell me all the things Leonora did to teach the children, and all she accomplished with the people here has inspired me," Opal continued, her face gleaming with enthusiasm.

"She's only been gone from the mission for about two years now," Flora added. "She became a wonderful friend to me during her time here. I sure do miss her."

Etta listened quietly as Flora told her about Leonora's adventures at the mission school. Little did they realize that a best-selling book would be written about this fascinating young woman, called <u>Christy</u>, nor did they have any way of knowing that some day television would be invented and <u>Christy</u> would become a popular TV series about Leonora's life in these mountains. To them Leonora was just someone who had reached out to help, just as a lot of other mountain people did when they were needed by their mountain neighbors.

Aunt Margaret Haney (everyone called her Aunt) was called to be the midwife for the delivery of Etta's second baby. Aunt Margaret was "blind as a bat." She had to have someone lead her around or she bumped into things, but she was still known to be one of the best midwives in the county. On November 29, 1919, Etta went into labor. Aunt Margaret used her hands to feel the baby's head and to tell how far along Etta was into labor. When the baby came, Aunt Margaret caught it, turned it up by its heels, and with a smack to its bottom, the baby began to cry. She laid the baby on the bed between Etta's legs while she took up the cord. Pushing the blood from the cord up toward the baby, she felt about how far to tie the cord, then she cut it. She then felt for the afterbirth, which was later taken up in the woods and buried. After cleaning the baby up, Aunt Margaret put the new addition to the Nichols family in Etta's arms. Harrison and Etta named their little bundle of joy Bessie June Nichols.

Two and a half years later, Etta became pregnant with her third child. During a visit with her mother, Etta shared the news with her family. Before she left, Novie told Etta about Furman's recent encounter with the measles. Novie was laughing so hard she could hardly tell the story. "Well, Furman had been sick with the red measles (German measles) fer several days," Novie said grinning widely, "but they wouldn't break out on 'im. So I told Lurlie to go down to the field and fetch me some sheep manure. I boiled the manure and strained the "tea" into a glass. Then I added some spices and sugar to it to cover up the taste of the manure. Ye know that's how ye get the measles to break out on the skin, don't ye?" Novie asked Etta.

Etta's face turned red as she giggled, "Well, I knowed about it, but I never have actually seed anybody use it."

"I took the tea to Furman and told him to drink it. He took a sip and said it tasted good. So he turned up the whole glass and swallered ever drop of it. I told him what it was a day or two after that. You should have seen his face, Etter! He looked like he hated the whole world. He told me I had caused him to lose his faith in people. He said he'd never trust anybody agin! I reminded him that the brew worked, fer thar weren't narry a spot on that child that wasn't broke out with the measles 30 minutes after he drunk that stuff. But he's still puffed up at me over that."

Etta stood beside her mother, her body shaking in laughter, as she pictured her little brother and the ordeal he had gone through. "Well, Mommie, it's getting late. It'll be 'bout dark before I get home if I don't leave now," Etta said. She gathered her belongings and said her goodbyes then started the long walk back to her farmhouse on the Huff Estate. Etta left the children at home with Harrison because they were still too young to travel such a long distance with her.

Etta quickly walked the beaten-down trails that wound through the thick forest land leading to her home; one hill, then another. She had walked among these woods by herself many times without fear, but this time she felt as if someone, or something, was following her. She quickened her pace. She could hear the leaves crackle behind her. "Dare I look around to identify my stalker?" she thought to herself. "No. Whatever it is might scare me so bad I'd fall down and be caught fer sure," Etta concluded as she began to run. Home was just over the top of the hill. She felt relief flow through her body at the sight of her house which was now in view. "Harrison! Harrison!" Etta shouted as she ran up the front yard. Harrison came out on the front porch to see what Etta's shouting was about. "Get your gun! Somethin' wuz followin' me through the woods," Etta told Harrison as she struggled to catch her breath. Harrison ran inside to retrieve his rifle. He stood on the porch for some time, but nothing appeared from the woods. Etta never did know what was following her in the woods, but a couple of days later one of her neighbors killed a panther while it was attempting to kill some of his livestock. It made Etta shiver to think it may have been the panther stalking her. Panthers usually lived higher up on the mountain, but occasionally one would come down looking for food at the foot of the mountain. "Thank you, God, fer watchin' over me," Etta whispered in silent prayer.

Carrie Buxton was a black lady who lived up a little dirt side road off the Midway section of Del Rio. She made her living by doing laundry for people in the community. When she returned the laundry to her customers it would be as white as snow. She was the only black person the mountain people would allow to live in their community. The road on which she lived was named "Nigger Branch" and would carry that name from then on. The people meant no disrespect to Carrie with the name they chose for the road, it was just that "nigger" was the only word any of the mountain people had ever

Etta "Granny" Nichols—Last of the Old-Timey Midwives

heard a black person called. Everyone liked Carrie and praised her work. Novie sent some laundry to Carrie each week because there was just too much for her to do alone.

When the time got closer for Etta to have her third baby, she went to stay with her mother so her family could help her with Emily and June. On April 11, 1923, John Lewis delivered his grandson. He was named Jasper Lewis Nichols; they would call him Jack. After Etta regained her strength, she and the children went back to their home on The Nathan Huff Estate.

A year passed and Jack was starting to walk. Harrison and Etta's house sat on a big, high bank which dropped off suddenly at one side of the yard. When Etta hung her laundry out to dry she took one end of a rope and tied it around Jack then tied the other end to a tree so he would not wander off and fall off the bank.

Etta stared teaching June how to do the dishes and help with the housework at the age of four, just as her mother had taught her at that age. Emily was now six years old. She did most of the housework, but she was sick a lot as a child, so when she could not do it, it was done by June. June also was sent to the tobacco fields to help pull weeds and hoe the crop at age four. Times were hard and Harrison could not afford to hire help in the fields. It would be up to the children to help their father.

Etta was visiting her mother and father when Earl Hann came riding up on his horse in an excited frenzy. He jumped from his horse and ran hurriedly up the steps on the front porch. John Lewis met him at the door to see what all the excitement was about.

"Doc, I think you ought'a go down to your daddy's house! I believe he's been killed," Earl said in a frantic voice.

John Lewis broke free from the shock that gripped his entire being after hearing the words which came from Earl's lips. He quickly ran to saddle his horse. Novie stood beside Etta with her hand over her mouth in disbelief as Earl and John Lewis rode off together. J. B. lived in the Slabtown community about a mile from John Lewis' house. Upon their arrival at J. B.'s house, Earl took John Lewis to his father, who was lying on the ground behind his house. He had been shot in the back with a .22 bullet. It was too late; J. B. was dead. John Lewis knew who had shot his father, but nobody would talk. He had the whole family arrested, but never had enough proof to keep them behind bars. They were released and John Lewis just had to let it go.

J. B. Grigsby died at age 78. He was buried in the family cemetery beside his wife, Rebecca, who had died the previous year on April 8, 1923.

Now that John Lewis was the only country doctor close by, he started getting called upon quite frequently. He would return home after seeing a patient with a ham, or chickens, or with whatever the people had, to pay him for his services. Sometimes he brought back money, but very rarely. Novie got angry with John Lewis for not insisting the people pay with cash, but John Lewis was an easygoing man who realized the poor people in the mountains needed what little money they had. He never did insist on being paid with money from anyone; he accepted whatever the families had to offer him.

John Lewis' Uncle Wiley had moved back to Tennessee from Molson, Washington in the Spring of 1921. He married Sarah Ann (Sallie) Sexton Sorrell, widow of John H. Sorrell. Wiley and Sallie owned and operated a general merchandise store in Slabtown. Wiley came up to John Lewis' house every year and helped him kill beef for the winter. Furman always looked forward to seeing his Great-uncle Wiley. He liked to listen to his wild tales and adventurous stories.

"If you want to kill a beef, you have'ta shoot it right thar," Wiley told Furman, pointing between his eyes.

John Lewis shook his head in agreement as the two men loaded their guns to prepare for the slaughter. BANG! A perfect shot. The cow fell to the ground. After skinning the cow the meat was placed in salt barrels to preserve it, then it was hung in the smokehouse until it was needed for a meal.

At Christmas time, Furman was having trouble believing that a big, fat man in a red suit came down his chimney to reward him each year for being a good boy. Novie decided she would have some fun with Furman this year. Harrison, Etta, and the children came to spend Christmas with Etta's family this year. On Christmas Eve Novie sent Harrison up on top of the house by the chimney. They used the wood stove in the kitchen to keep warm on this particular night. After all, one could not expect Santa Claus to come down a chimney that had a fire burning in it! Novie told the children to gather around in the front room. She held her apron up under the opening of the chimney and said, "Okay, Santa Claus, roll me down about a dozen apples." Harrison tossed down the apples from the top of the chimney. Furman about had a "duck fit"! It scared him half to death. J. L. ran over and grabbed Etta's dress tail and would not let go until they calmed him down. John Lewis had been on a house call and had come in just after the children's frightful encounter with Santa Claus.

"You kids get on up to bed so Santa Claus can deliver the rest of your presents," John Lewis ordered the children. The children did as their father instructed without hesitation. "Now you can make a kid grow up nervous and have trouble later on doin' such foolishness as that. I don't ever want you to do anythang like that agin!" John scolded Novie.

Furman still was not convinced that Santa was real. He got out of bed and snuck to the stairs. He quietly peeped around the corner and watched as Novie filled each stocking hanging over the mantel with two oranges, a handful of English walnuts, pecans, Brazil nuts, and a peppermint candy cane one and a half feet long by two inches wide. Now Furman knew for sure who Santa really was.

On Christmas morning all the children sprang from their beds in a frenzy to get to their stockings. The fruit, nuts, and candy was a big treat for them. This was the only time of the year they got to eat such delightful yummies. After everyone had settled down from their excitement Furman approached his mother with a crafty look on his face.

"Now I know who Santa Claus is," Furman said with aplomb.

Novie looked down at Furman in surprise. "How 'da ye know that?"

"I watched you and Daddy fill the stockin's last night," replied Furman.

Novie became terribly upset with Furman for sneaking out of his bed, but she did not punish him because it was Christmas.

A big breakfast of 15 eggs fried in hog lard, ham, and about 20 biscuits and gravy started off the day. A huge Christmas dinner was always prepared in the afternoon. A wild turkey was killed and dressed by John Lewis and Waitsel, while Novie and Etta prepared Chicken n' dumplings, chicken dressing, green beans, corn on the cob, cornbread, and buttermilk for the Christmas feast. Before eating, family members bowed their heads and said a silent blessing over the food, then the bowls were passed from one person to the next until their plates had no more room left on them. For dessert Etta made a stack cake which was totally consumed by the family. After the delicious Christmas dinner was over everyone settled in close to the fire and took a well-deserved nap.

The winter months passed slowly. John Lewis would come home many nights with icicles in his two-day beard. He would travel as far as North Carolina to treat the sick. He was said to be the best doctor around for treating fevers. There were times when he would go into a home and find five to ten people all sick in bed. He would treat each one, staying as long as he was needed, until they were well enough to do for themselves.

Etta loved to listen to her father's stories about his journeys across the mountains and what he used to treat his patients. She still wanted to be a nurse with all of her heart, but she feared her dream would never come true. Harrison and Etta were poor, and she had little children of her own to raise now. Going to school to learn nursing was totally out of the question.

At the age of 15, Willie (Bill), Etta's youngest sister, caught a disease called scrofula. It made her lymph nodes in her neck swell and affected her vocal cords and hearing. Afterward, Willie had to read lips in order to tell what was being said, and it was hard for her to speak. She was a beautiful young woman with blond hair, blue eyes, and a fair complexion. She would not let the loss of her hearing or voice discourage her; she would go on to lead a fulfilling life in spite of her disabilities.

Spring came; it was time to plant crops and work in the fields and gardens once more. Each year was pretty much the same for the farmers, unless the weather did not cooperate. Sometimes many weeks would pass with no rain. During the droughts the men had to hand-carry buckets of water to the crops from the creek. Sometimes the field was a great distance from the creek. Other times hailstorms would beat down the crops until nothing was worth saving. But during hard times such as these, neighbor helped neighbor, and that was something all the people of the Appalachian Mountains could count on.

Novie was now 48 and expecting her eleventh child. It was a harsh pregnancy for her because of her age. She and John Lewis started experiencing problems in their marriage. Novie was not willing to compromise at all. She was even more stubborn now than when they had first married, and no one was going to change her; John Lewis still possessed his easygoing temperament.

When the time came for the baby to be born, John Lewis assisted his wife, but the baby was stillborn. Novie was going through "the change of life" during this pregnancy, which sadly was a determinant in the fate of the child. The baby boy was buried in the Grigsby Cemetery with his brothers and grandparents. He was not given a name and no marker was placed on his grave.

A couple of months passed and Novie had regained all her strength. Furman was down at the creek, a "far piece" from the house, catching horny heads. Novie and Etta were in the house visiting together. Furman suddenly heard a terrifying noise coming up the road. He looked up and dirt was rolling off the side of the road above him. He threw down his fishing rod in a panic and placed a large rock on top of the fish he had already caught to prevent them from flopping back into the water. At age 10 a child can be frightened quite easily by the unknown. Furman took off running in a panic in his knee pants and bare feet toward the house, but he took a short-cut through the briar patch in order to get there quicker. When he came bursting through the door his legs were bloody all over. Novie looked at him and in a baffled voice asked, "What on earth have you been a doin'? You're as bloody as a hog!"

Furman answered while trying to catch his breath, "Mommie, I want you to listen to what's a-comin' up the road!"

About that time Novie heard the racket coming closer and closer. She walked over to the window and gasped in disbelief as she exclaimed, "They, Lord have mercy! Is the end of time a-comin'? Look a-comin' yonder!!"

Seeing the fear on his mother's face, Furman ran to a pile of dirty clothes on the floor and he crawled under them to hide. Etta hurried to the window to see what in the world was going on. Dirt was rolling off the sides of the road and the sound terrified Novie and Etta as they viewed a huge orange monster plowing its way up the road in front of the house. It was Chub Moore on a road scraper smoothing out the road. Neither Novie nor Etta had ever witnessed such a thing in all their life! This would be a day neither of them would ever forget. Thirty minutes passed before Novie realized she had not seen Furman around anywhere. She and Etta looked for some time before they finally found him shaking under the pile of dirty clothes. It took awhile, but all three finally composed themselves after the horrifying experience, and Furman went back to the creek to finish his fishing.

John Lewis returned home one evening with news that he had found a buyer for the sawmill and all his land in Meadows Field. He had been trying for years to raise the money to pay off George Runnion, and now he could finally do it. After getting all the paperwork in order, John Lewis sold his land to Joe Smith and paid off his debt. He bought about an acre of land from Zack Messer down the road about a half a mile from where they lived in Meadows Field. It was across the creek from some other land Joe Smith owned. This area in the community was known as London, named by John Lewis' father, J. B. Grigsby. The land had a small wooden house located on it. A mud-daubed chimney rose from the ground to above the roof on the left side of the structure. The sound of the creek located at the edge of the front yard could be heard while relaxing on the front porch. A green field stretched out on the other side of the creek harmonized with the swaying of the tall, tranquil trees on the small mountain at the field's edge. This was now the Grigsby family's new home.

Novie was very upset that she and John Lewis only had $400 left after paying George Runnion and buying the land in London. She quarreled with John Lewis more and more. It seemed to him he could not do anything to please his wife anymore. Novie felt John Lewis' dream of owning a sawmill had cost them too much and she stared to resent John Lewis.

As winter approached, John Lewis was staying away on house calls as much as he could to avoid Novie's nasty temper. John had a horse named Nell. That horse was John Lewis' only companion during his days of travel across the mountains. She was smart, too—if John Lewis started to lean to one side in the saddle, being weary from a long journey, Nell would lean over the opposite direction to put him back straight in the saddle. One bitterly cold night, after everyone was in bed, John Lewis came riding home on good ol' Nell. His feet were frozen to the stirrups on the saddle, preventing him from dismounting. Icicles were frozen on his three-day beard; he was almost frozen to death. He could not call out to his family for help. Nell sensed her master needed help. She stepped up to the porch and pawed the wooden steps loudly until someone came out. Lurlie and Furman came out and knocked their father's feet loose from the icy stirrups. Nell leaned way over to allow the boys to get a hold of John Lewis. They helped their father to the fireplace where he lay thawing out for quite awhile before he was able to move freely. Nell remained with John Lewis until her death, a loyal friend and companion.

• • • • • •

Harrison learned of some farm land at Blue Mill he could rent from the government for $12 a year. It already had a little three-room house on it where they could live. Jim Crowder came with a big truck to help Harrison and Etta move. It was dark before they got the truck loaded. Jim got in and started the engine only to find out the headlights would not burn. He got out of the truck, raised the hood, and walked around to Etta. "Would you happen to have a stick of gum on you, Etta?" Jim asked.

Etta wanted him to get back under the hood and fix the problem, but she reluctantly pulled out a piece of peppermint gum from her hand-sewn brown apron. "Here you go. I just happened to have a stick in my apron," Etta answered as she handed the gum to Jim.

Jim took the gum out and gave it to Emily. Now Etta was really confused as to why Jim asked for the stick of gum. Jim took the foil wrapper and wrapped it around the fuse going to the headlights. He walked confidently back to get inside the truck. He started the engine once more, pulled the knob to turn on the headlights, and instantly they came on. Etta thought that little trick was amazing. She told that story to everyone she saw for the longest time. With everyone loaded inside the vehicle, the Nichols family was anxious to get started on the journey to their new home. As the passenger door slammed shut, June let out a scream that would curl straight hair. Someone had mashed her fingers in the door. Etta examined them, making sure nothing was broken. After some time consoling her, June's cries subsided and the 10-mile ride began.

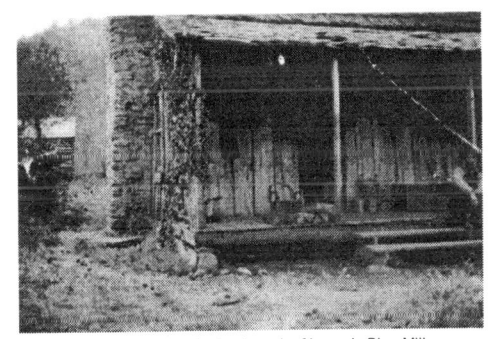

Upon Harrison and Etta's arrival in Blue Mill the little bit of furniture they owned was unloaded from the truck, along with clothes, dishes, pots and pans, quilts, pillows, a cedar chest, and other items. They placed a full-size bed in the front room, along with a dresser and another half-size bed. A large fireplace occupied one side of the wall. The kitchen was long and spacious. The other room would be used for a bedroom for the girls. The walls were covered with funny papers from the local newspaper throughout the house to help insulate it from the heat and cold outside. The house set in a big open field with plenty of room for the kids to play without Etta having

Harrison sits on the front porch of home in Blue Mill

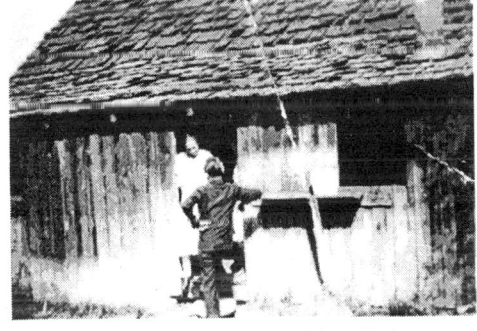

Etta talks to a neighbor from the back door of the house.

to worry about one of them falling off the bank, as she did while living on The Huff Estate.

A bubbling, clear water creek ran in front of the house just in the distance. Across the creek was Lonnie Moore's general store where a person could purchase sugar, flour, meal, candy, and other necessities. A large mill occupied the space to the left of the store. Meal and flour were ground from corn and sold in the store. Local farmers could also bring their corn and crops for grinding to the mill.

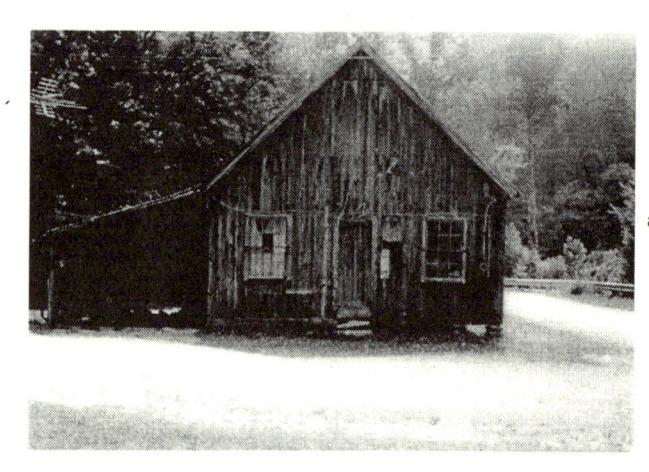

Lonnie Moore's store as it appeared in 1996

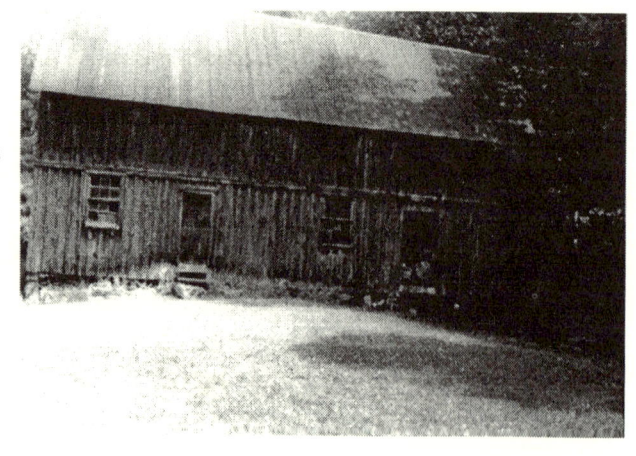

The water mill as it appeared in 1996

Etta "Granny" Nichols—Last of the Old-Timey Midwives

Steep mountains, just starting to bud with the first signs of spring, enclosed the area on each side of the open meadow where the house set. A narrow foot-log provided the only path over the rippling creek from the house to the other side leading to Lonnie's store. The foot-log would be traveled upon quite frequently by the new residents of Blue Mill.

Easter was an exciting time for Emily and June. They gathered green walnut hulls from the ground and boiled them in water to produce a green dye for their eggs. They also wet different colors of crepe paper to wrap around the eggs. Except for the time spent in church, the children spent most of the day hiding eggs. Etta seemed to associate Easter with eggs, as well, except hers appeared scrambled on the kitchen table...for all three meals of the day. She did this each year on Easter Sunday.

Church was attended three times a day each Sunday. The family walked across two or three big mountains to attend church at Oak Grove. Afternoon and night service was attended at Mulberry Gap, just up the road about three fourths of a mile.

The Mulberry Gap church was used as a school during the week for all the children who could attend. June appreciated the school being so close to her new home. She no longer had to walk for miles through the spooky woods or encounter the bullies who tried to scare her with their horse on her way to school. Several boys, all from the same family, would act like they were going to run over her, and June would have to run behind a tree to hide. One of the boy's would yell, "Come out from behind that tree so we can see ye. We won't hurt ye if we can see ye." June would stay put until the boys rode away. She would be so nervous by the time she got to school, she could not concentrate on her studies.

"Maybe now I can calm my nerves and do better in school," June thought to herself.

Each day after school June and Jack were sent to the woods to cut down a tree for firewood for the cookstove. The children struggled with the cumbersome limbs as they dragged the tree through the forest to their backyard. There they sawed it with Harrison's hand saw into small logs so they would fit easily into the wood stove. After the wood was gathered and stacked up by the fireplace they had to find the milk cow and bring her to the barn to be milked. She could be anywhere on the mountain. Sometimes finding her was a chore in itself. After milking the cow and bringing the full bucket of milk back to the kitchen, the milk was strained through a clean white cloth and poured into crocks. They carried the crocks to the spring house, where it was placed in the cold water to keep it cool and fresh-tasting. After the milking, the children carried water from the spring and filled the water buckets in the house to ensure enough water would be on hand for the following day. Emily usually tended to most of the chores inside the house. After all the chores were done, Emily and June gathered up dirty clothes and tied them together to make a ragdoll to play with. The children had to use whatever they could for entertainment; real toys were scarce and too expensive to buy.

Etta was expecting her fourth child when they moved to Blue Mill. She sent Harrison after her father, who lived about a mile away from their new home, to come deliver

Etta "Granny" Nichols—Last of the Old-Timey Midwives

his grandchild. John Lewis arrived soon after on his horse, Nell. He told the children to stay outside with their father as he entered the house and walked over to where Etta was lying on the bed. Several hours passed before a cuddly little redheaded girl emerged to make her claim as the newest member of the Nichols family. Born on May 2, 1929, she was named Margaret Verta Lula Belle Nichols, after her four aunts, although Margaret Belle Nichols was all that was entered on her birth certificate.

Harrison made a deal with Stokely Brothers in Newport to raise tomatoes for their canning factory. He and June spent many days going to the tomato patch up in Rocky Holler to plow and pull weeds. Harrison hoed the row while June pulled weeds from the middle. He was afraid she might mistake a tomato plant for a weed if she got too close to the plants. One day as Harrison and June were working in the tomatoes, LaFayette Moore came walking across the hill. He stopped and looked over the budding tomato plants with a grin on his face. "I know whur I can git me some 'maters at this summer," he said, grinning.

Harrison leaned up on the end of his hoe and said boldly, "There might be a shotgun up here, too."

"Oh, I won't bother it," LaFayette replied through a mischievous smile.

Harrison got tickled at LaFayette's remark. He always was a big cutup with everybody.

Harrison and LaFayette talked a few minutes, then LaFayette hurried on over the hill to his destination. This would be the only year Harrison would raise a tomato crop. It was very time-consuming and he needed more help than he had. He would stick to raising tobacco and corn in the years to come.

The hot summer months passed and fall arrived. In October 1929, the stock market crashed, the economy fell to an all-time low. The bank in Newport closed its doors. Anyone having money in the bank lost their savings—for some it was their life savings. Big businesses were suddenly bankrupt. One in four workers lost jobs. Others lost their homes because they could not pay the mortgage. Many families had no money to buy food. In the larger cities people stood in line for food. People started to panic; some committed suicide. The economic devastation was felt even in the mountains of Del Rio, but people there were already used to hard times, so they would fare better than people living in the cities. They had their gardens to grow vegetables and fruit, chickens to lay eggs, cows to provide milk, and hogs and beef to kill for meat. The Great Depression left its mark on everyone, but the people of the Appalachian Mountains would survive the difficult years ahead.

PART III

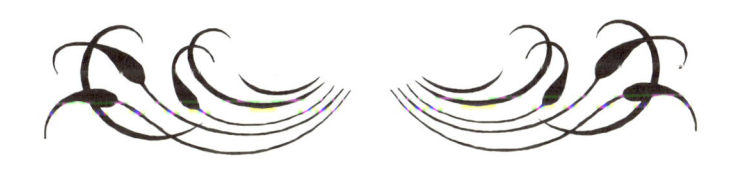

The Birth Of A New Midwife

PART III

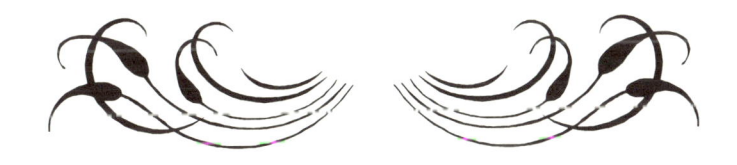

The Birth Of A New Midwife

The long harsh winter of 1929 was over. Etta celebrated her 33rd birthday on May 19th. She had four children to raise and a loving husband who worked hard to provide for his family. Emily would turn 13 in July; June would be 11 in November; Jack turned 7 in April, and Belle turned 1 in May.

One afternoon as Etta was walking home from her mother's, her children in a half-run trying to keep up with her, she met Edatha Morrow's brother hurrying to her father's house to get him to come and deliver his sister's baby. "He ain't home right now," Etta told the man.

"Will you go up there?" the man asked in a panic.

Etta had experience in delivering babies from going out with her father on "baby cases." She had never delivered a baby by herself, but she was not afraid. She agreed to go help Edatha who lived up the road from her house in Norwood Town. She quickly sent the children to the field to get Harrison to come stay with them as they approached their house. When Harrison came she took off up the road going as fast as her legs would carry her. When she arrived, Edatha was lying in bed. Etta washed her hands in the hottest water she could stand. She then told Edatha she needed to check her to see how far in labor she was. Etta felt the baby's head. She told Edatha, "I can feel its head. Stand up a little bit and see if your water will break." Edatha did as Etta requested. It was not long until her water broke. She laid back down on the bed and held Etta's hands as she stared bearing down with the pains. "Here it comes!" Etta said excitedly. She got hold of the baby's shoulders and helped pull it out. "It's a boy!" Etta told the proud new mother. She cut the cord and cleaned the baby up. She put a white cloth diaper on him then wrapped him in a soft cotton blanket before putting him in his mother's arms. Edatha named her little newcomer Bud. Etta then helped Edatha get cleaned up. Edatha's mother and Etta took the afterbirth up the road and buried it. With mother and baby doing fine, Etta collected a $2 fee for her services then headed back home. She was exhilarated with what she had just experienced. Her first delivery was a success. Little did she realize that there would be over 2,000 more deliveries for her to attend to in the future.

It did not take long for the word to spread about the new midwife in the mountains. Etta was "goin' first one place and then another" delivering babies throughout the mountains. People came after Etta sometimes when the pain was not really severe, and she would stay two or three days until the real labor started. She left her children in Harrison's care. He was home every day anyway, being a farmer. Belle stood on the front porch and cried for her mother when she stayed gone for long periods of time. Emily and June were responsible for the household chores which their mother usually took care of, along with their regular chores, until Etta returned home. Jack helped his father in the garden, cornfield, and tobacco patch.

It was January 13, 1932, when Ance Lunsford knocked on Etta's door.

"Mrs. Nichols, could you come to my house? My wife is 'bout to have the baby," Ance asked nervously.

"I sure can. Just let me get my things," Etta answered. "Emily, you watch Belle 'til I get back." Etta put on her long wool coat and wrapped a thick cotton scarf over her head before she and Ance started walking up the road. Ance and his wife, Ethel Carlisle Lunsford, lived about 3/4 of a mile up the dirt road from Harrison and Etta. The air was cold and crisp, as it blew gently through the barren trees. The fast pace at which Etta and Ance walked helped to keep them warm. Upon Etta's arrival at the Lunsford home, she quickly washed her hands in hot water, then she checked Ethel.

"Well, it looks like I got here just in time," Etta told Ethel. "This baby is ready to see the world," Etta giggled. "The next time you get a strong 'misery' I want you to push with all your strength." Ethel let out a scream as the baby's head started coming through. "One more time, Ethel! It's here—just give one more good push."

Ance heard the baby let out its first cry as he waited anxiously in the front room. He immediately went to the bedroom to check on his wife and meet his new baby.

"It's a girl," Etta told Ance as he entered the bedroom.

"Isn't she beautiful," Ethel said looking up at her proud husband. Ance nodded his head in agreement.

"What'er you gonna name 'er?" Etta asked.

"Audrey...Audrey Lunsford," replied Ethel.

"Well, you be sure to tell Audrey that she's the first baby girl that I ever helped deliver when she grows up, okay?"

"Is that a fact?!" replied Ance. "Yeah, we'll be sure to tell 'er all 'bout you—how you helped us fer nothin', and what a fine lady you are."

"Well, I'd better head back home now. If you need me fer anything, just holler," Etta said as she put on her coat and head scarf. Etta knew how poor this couple was, so she never asked for any kind of payment. She felt a stronger, different kind of payment inside her heart. The feeling she received every time she helped bring a new life into the world was payment enough for her.

After going on several more baby cases, Etta decided she needed a little black medical bag like her dad used. She kept clean white rags, nitrate drops to put in the newborn's eyes, and some ergot to help with contractions during labor. She also used quinine to help reduce fever when necessary. Castor oil was administered only if the patient was ready to go into labor, otherwise it would not work on starting the labor pains. Etta never used any kind of painkillers; she believed a woman should be alert and not drugged during childbirth. Also, in her little black bag she kept the birth certificates which were filled out on each baby after its birth. Tim Monroe, the mail carrier, picked up the certificates in Etta's mailbox and delivered them to the U.S. Post Office along the railroad tracks just before coming to the French Broad River in Del Rio. From there the documents were sent to the Health Department in Newport, and from there they were sent to Nashville to be filed.

Emily, June, and Jack did what they could to help earn money. They spent countless evenings picking up walnuts to sell. They had to crack them and have them free of any hull before sending them to the marketplace.

June helped the neighbors hoe corn. She helped Mrs. Stinson hoe corn all day long and was paid 50 cents for her labor. She spent her money purchasing material from the Sears and Roebuck catalog to sew herself a new dress, or to buy a new pair of shoes. Sometimes the shoes she ordered would be too small, but she kept them anyway because she needed them so badly. She developed terrible corns on her toes because her shoes were too small, but all the children considered a new pair of shoes a blessing whether they fit properly or not.

Etta sewed most of the clothes the younger children wore on her treadle Singer sewing machine. She pumped the wide metal foot pedal to control the speed of the needle, they did not have electricity in the mountains of Del Rio.

Etta sold eggs to Lonnie Moore at his store across the creek from her house for small change, or sometimes she traded them for other items she needed in the kitchen. Almost everything they ate was raised in their garden. They had green beans, potatoes, corn, tomatoes, cucumbers, squash, and pumpkins. An apple tree provided the necessary fruit for Etta to make her delicious apple pies, and a large grapevine in the back yard produced numerous ripe, juicy grapes. Belle crawled under the vines and ate grapes until her belly was full each summer. Etta made a tasty grape jelly as an extra treat for her family. In the latter part of summer Etta and the children always went blackberry picking. The mountains were full of blackberry patches, but one had to be very careful because blackberries were not the only thing the woods were full of. There were moonshine stills all through the hills. If a person happened to come upon one during his travels he might be surprised by a shotgun staring him in the face. After the blackberries were gathered, Etta made blackberry dumplings, blackberry jam, and blackberry pies. Wild strawberries grew plentifully throughout the mountains also. They were gathered about the same time as the blackberries. Strawberries with milk or cream was a favorite of all the family. Strawberry jam was made with any leftover berries.

Breakfast usually consisted of eggs with sausage or bacon, gravy, and biscuits. The noonday meal was always the most important meal of the day. It would be the only meal Etta would cook for the rest of the day. Any leftovers were left on the table and covered with a cotton table cloth for the family to snack on during the rest of the day. There was no way to preserve food; once it was cooked, it had to be eaten. The evening meal was always cornbread and milk...every day of every week.

On Sundays the noonday meal was typically fried chicken, or chicken and dumplings. Harrison went outside with Etta to pick out the chicken that would be on the kitchen table for the family's Sunday dinner. Once Etta pointed out the bird of her choice, Harrison grabbed the chicken by the neck and slung it around and around, breaking its neck. The bird flopped around on the ground until it was dead. Harrison then plucked all the feathers off and gave it to Etta. She cleaned the chicken in a big round dishpan and cut it up for the frying pan, which contained melted hog lard. After rolling the chicken in flour, adding salt and pepper, the chicken was placed in the frying pan, sending an aroma throughout the house that made ones mouth water. During the meal the children took turns standing over the table with a long stick, which had strips of newspaper sewed onto it at the end, fanning the table to keep flies off the food while the rest of the family ate; the windows had no screens to keep the pests out of the house during the hot summer months.

The winter months arrived, making travel very difficult for Etta, but she never turned anyone away who needed her. She had been known to walk 8-10 miles with snow almost to her knees and back home again, the cold bitter wind chapping her cherry-colored cheeks. The last house call she went on was a little risky; the baby was turned wrong, with the feet coming out first. Etta told the woman to get on her knees and raise her rear as high in the air as she could. After holding that position for about 10 or 15 minutes, the baby turned so the head was coming out first. Etta's father had taught her how to handle breech babies, which he had encountered several times. The mother and baby were both fine. Etta always told the mother, should the baby develop colic, to give it goat's milk, but she recommended the mother breast-feed the baby above anything else if the baby was not colicky. Sometimes she was paid with eggs, chickens, or a slab of beef. She received her $2 fee in cash from time to time. Sometimes the people were just too poor to pay her with anything, but she never turned anyone away because they could not afford to pay her.

Belle snuggled in bed between her mother and father at night in the front room. Jack, Emily, and June shared the other bedroom. They slept on straw-tick mattresses, which had to be fluffed up each morning when making the beds. When the fire went out during the night the house became bitterly cold. Layers of homemade quilts lay on top of one another to keep the children warm.

Everyone was expected to rise early each morning. Six o'clock was considered late to be getting out of bed. Harrison was the first one to get up. He started the fire burning in the fireplace in the front room, and also in the wood stove in the kitchen so it would be ready for Etta to cook breakfast. Belle snuggled up close to her mother's warm breast until the rooms were heated. Etta then got up and started the sausage, eggs, gravy, and biscuits until

Emily, June, and Jack were awakened by the wonderful aroma.

Harrison always called Belle "Baby Girl." He called to her from the kitchen each morning, "Get up, Baby Girl."

"Come 'n get me," Belle would answer in a petted tone.

Harrison retrieved her from the bed and carried her to the chair in front of the fireplace and put her clothes on her. She wore long underwear with thick white cotton stockings reaching the top of her thighs to keep her legs warm, and a little white dress with long sleeves. Jack wore patched overalls with a long-sleeved cotton shirt underneath; Emily and June both wore dresses with thick white cotton stockings. It was considered a sin for a woman to wear pants or shorts.

After doing their morning chores, June and Jack walked to school at Mulberry Gap. Emily stayed home and helped her mother with the household chores. She watched Belle while Etta and Harrison tended to the morning milking. The crocks of strained milk were covered with white cloths and plates set on top to hold them in place. When the cream rose to the top of the crock it was skimmed off and taken to the churn to make butter and buttermilk. Sometimes there would not be as much cream as Etta thought there should be. She did not realize Belle had been sneaking to the spring house with a spoon and eating most of the cream before she collected it for the churn. Etta and Emily took turns sitting with the churn. It had a wooden handle with wooden extensions that fit into the crock to churn the butter. Emily sat until her arm was in pain from the up-and-down motion needed to make the butter. Once the butter was ready, it was removed and placed into a butter mold. On the top of the butter, after being removed from the mold, was a little flower imprinted into the butter. Each mold of butter weighed about one pound and could be sold at the store. The milk left in the crock became the best-tasting buttermilk in the mountains. Etta loved her buttermilk, and that was a fact!

Another winter had passed. The wild flowers sprouted in splendor all over the open fields. The trees that had been bare for so long now painted the mountains shades of light green, while the pine trees cast a darker shade of green, giving definition to the boastful Round Mountain. It could be seen just up the road from Harrison and Etta's house. Further down the road, where Etta's great-grandfather had lived, one could view Max Patch, one of the taller peaks in the eastern end of the Great Smoky Mountains. It had an altitude of 4,629 feet. The summit on Max Patch had 600 acres of grass land. No timber had ever grown there.

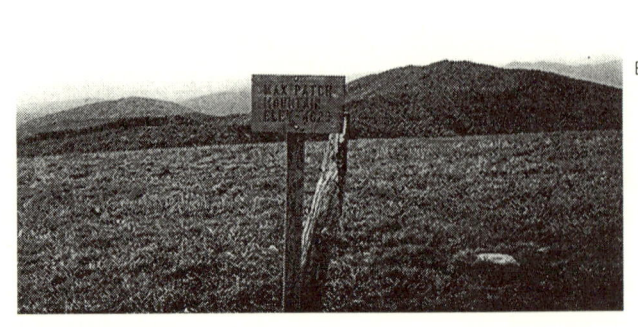

Max Patch Mountain—
Elevation - 4629

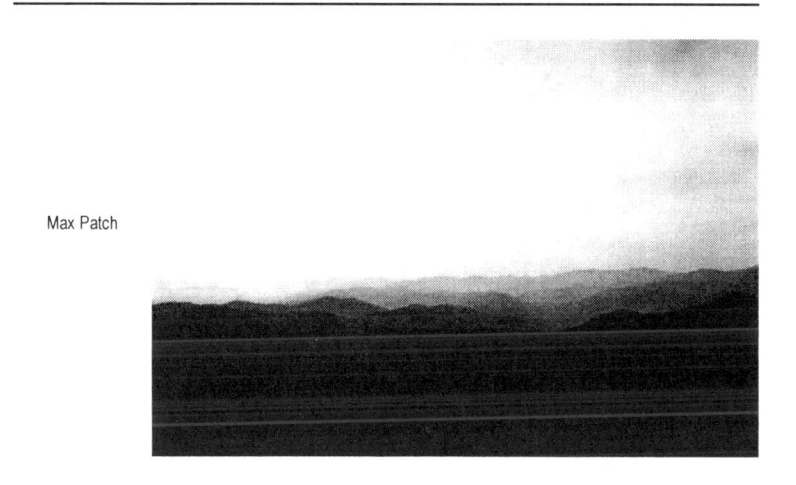

Etta "Granny" Nichols—Last of the Old-Timey Midwives

Max Patch

From Del Rio one could see the fields of Max Patch were still covered in a protective blanket of white snow, which glistened in the bright sunlight. Etta had lived in other places, but none could compare to her home in the beautiful mountains of East Tennessee. This was where her heart called "home," and she would never leave it again.

Another year passed, and Belle was now three and a half years old. She loved going over to Lonnie Moore's store. He spoiled her with candy each time she visited him. Belle loved going to the mill; the big water wheel fascinated her. Lonnie would pick her up and carry her up to the mill where she watched as the corn was ground by the huge water wheel which turned continuously, splashing up the water in the creek.

One day Etta was busy canning pickles when she discovered she was out of vinegar. She sent Belle to Lonnie's store to get her some. Belle crossed the narrow foot-log stretching across the creek and ran into the store. She stood there with a bewildered expression on her face as she tried to figure out how she would ask Lonnie for the vinegar, since she could not pronounce the word.

Lonnie stood tall beside Belle as he looked down and asked her. "What can I get for you, Little Lady?"

"Mama wants some of that sour stuff," Belle answered, straining her neck looking up at Lonnie.

Lonnie grinned widely at Belle's request. "I believe I know what you're talking about." He retrieved the bottle of vinegar from the shelf and handed it to Belle, along with a piece of candy and a wink. Belle hurried back home to give her mother the vinegar then she went out on the front porch where she sat enjoying her candy in the warm summer breeze.

Fall brought with it the harvesting season. The corn was picked from the stalk and put into bushel baskets. Some of the neighbors had corn shuckin's where all the neighbors gathered to lend a hand to one another. Teenagers used these gatherings to meet a potential boyfriend or girlfriend. They made a game out of their labor, seeing who could shuck the most corn in a given amount of time. June had her eye on Clyde Roberts. She had had a crush on him ever since she met him at church. He walked her home after service sometimes, Etta walking a short distance behind them.

June worked in the tobacco along with Harrison and Jack, helping to grade and tie it. It was then hung in the barn until it was ready to be shipped to the warehouse in Newport to be sold.

June often walked to Jim and Bertie Lamb's house to do laundry all day and then walk back home, about three miles, to earn 25 cents. One day while she was there

Bertie asked if she would like to ride to Newport with her and Jim. Carmel Seay drove a taxi from Del Rio to Newport, since not many people in Del Rio owned a car. They hired him to make the 20-mile journey there and back home. June was 13 but she had never been out of Del Rio. She was scared half to death as they approached the city; she had never seen such a big place with so many buildings and people. She held on to Bertie's dress as they walked through the store, afraid she would get lost in the crowd. After Bertie finished her business, she, Jim, and June returned to Carmel Seay's taxi to start back home. June was glad to be leaving and going back to the safety she felt in the wide-open country surrounding her home, but she was also glad she had made the journey to Newport. Just wait until she told her friends she had been to the city!

Lena Smith was another lady June did laundry for. Her house was a long way over the mountain. June scrubbed the clothes on a washboard using homemade lye soap. She would spend half a day there for 25 cents. She could not spend as much time there because it took her a long time to walk back home.

President Hoover had been voted out of office and was replaced with President Franklin D. Roosevelt. In his inaugural address, President Roosevelt called for faith in America's future. "The only thing we have to fear is fear itself," he declared boldly. He launched a program to help give aid to the average American he called, "the forgotten man." His program was called the "New Deal." He promised relief for unemployed workers and aid to farmers, and he started new government agencies to help, such as CCC, TVA, NRA, and WPA.

One of the relief programs started by President Roosevelt provided food to anyone in need of it. Surplus food was shipped monthly to Newport where it could be picked up by the locals for distribution. One of Harrison and Etta's neighbors made the monthly trip to Newport for several people in the Del Rio community, bringing back enough food to help them get through the month ahead. Large sacks of pinto beans, coffee, sugar, flour, meal, salt, and other food supplies was delivered to Etta's front porch each month.

President Roosevelt made good on his promise. His programs were helping to take some of the hardships off people which the Great Depression had placed upon them.

John Lewis was one of the first people in the Del Rio community to buy a car. It was a leather-top convertible Redbird Overland, which he purchased at Kyker's Auto Sales in Newport. Some of the residents in Del Rio were jealous of John Lewis' new vehicle. They snubbed up their noses as he drove by, displaying their feelings openly. John Lewis did not let it bother him. He knew he was well liked by most of the community.

Novie continued with her quarrelsome attitude towards John Lewis, until she finally told him she wanted a divorce. John Lewis pleaded with her to let him stay with her because they still had three young sons at home who needed their father—Lurlie, Furman, and J. L. (Waitsel had married Latha Ellen Clark on March 16, 1919. They settled on a plot of land in an area called Spicewood Flats, just a few miles up the road from where John Lewis and Novie lived; Willie had married Arthur Gowans and settled in North Carolina; Alvertie married Dallas Taylor and also had started a family of her own).

After seeing Novie was not going to give into his pleas, John Lewis agreed to give Novie a divorce, something very uncommon for people of their day. He gave Novie the house and the land in the divorce settlement, and he kept the car and his personal belongings. John Lewis packed his things and made arrangements to stay with his daughter Willie in North Carolina.

Etta was devastated by her parents' divorce. She felt loyalty to both her parents and was torn in different directions. Although she had her own family now, she was deeply saddened knowing her father would be so far away. She always looked forward to seeing him on her visits to their house, but now he would no longer be there.

John Lewis continued to make attempts, after he had moved out, to talk Novie into taking him back, but she would not. He missed his boys tremendously. After much discussion, John Lewis convinced Novie to let Furman come stay with him in North Carolina. Novie was having trouble keeping food in the house since John Lewis was no longer there. "One less mouth to feed might help out," she thought to herself.

After several months passed, John Lewis met Violet Payne in North Carolina. Later, after a brief courtship, they were married.

Novie was still having trouble feeding her two remaining sons living at home. J. L. would often walk up to Etta's and she would fix him a hearty meal and give him an apple pie to take home. Etta was looked upon as a mother figure instead of an older sister by all her siblings, since she was the one who had taken care of them when they were growing up.

• • • • • •

The year was 1936. Emily would be 19 years old in July; June would be 17 in November; Jack turned 13 in April, and Belle would be 7 in May.

At 13 Jack caught the mumps in one side of his jaw. He received a lot of extra attention from everyone at home, which made Belle jealous. She was the one used to getting all the attention, being the baby in the family. One morning when Etta and Harrison were in the kitchen, Belle crawled into bed with Jack in hopes of getting the mumps, too. She wanted the kind of attention he was getting. Her wish came true. Several days after coming in close contact to Jack, Belle's jaw began to swell. June also caught the contagious virus. Since June was older, the virus was worse for her than it had been for her younger brother and sister. Her jaws swelled so large she could barely open her mouth wide enough to get a knife between her teeth. She had to live on liquids for almost two weeks. Jack's case of mumps was getting better, he thought. He was tired of being confined to his bed, so he snuck outside to play. Poor Jack should not have done that, because it triggered the onset of the mumps in the other side of his jaw, and he was confined to his bed for another two weeks. Belle fared better than June and Jack because she was so young, but she also endured her fair share of pain. She would be more careful in the future as to what she wished for. Emily had moved in with a family in Newport, Fred and Emma Jones, so she avoided contracting the mumps from her siblings. Emily helped do the housework for a small wage and room and board.

On May 5, 1936, three days after Belle turned 7, Etta received word that her father had died. He had been sick for some time, suffering from stomach cancer, which led to his death one week shy of his 61st birthday. His body was brought back by horse and wagon from North Carolina to Del Rio where he was buried in the Mulberry Gap Cemetery. Etta would miss her father greatly. An emptiness filled her heart as she had never known before, but she would look to God, her Master, to give her the strength to deal with her loss.

Etta continued going on her baby cases all across the Appalachian Mountains. Now that Emily was no longer living at home, the housework was left up to June and Belle while their mother was gone. June not only had the housework to do, but she also helped in the fields. Jack also helped in the fields, but he often complained with a bellyache and Harrison would let him go home.

Belle and Jack walked to Mulberry Gap school each day. It was about three-fourths of a mile up the road from their house. Erdine Jones taught the class as the students sat on the long wooden benches which filled the classroom. Around lunchtime Etta would come walking up the dirt road carrying a large kettle of homemade vegetable soup to feed all the children at the school. She did this every day she was home. The families of the children attending the school all donated the vegetables for Etta to prepare the soup. It contained mostly potatoes, onions, and tomatoes seasoned with salt and pepper, but to the hungry children, Etta's homemade vegetable soup was delectable.

Ola Moore was looking for a companion to keep her company, since she lived all alone, except for her young daughter. Her husband had to leave the area to work on his job. June heard about her search and pleaded with her mother and daddy to let her go live with the woman. It would be a way for her to earn some extra money. Harrison and Etta agreed to let June go. Mrs. Moore lived about one and a half miles up the road from them, so it was not as if June would be out of touch. Mrs. Moore lived in a small three-room wooden house guarded by a mean dog, which tried to bite anyone who came on her place. Belle went up there with June once, and the dog acted as if it was going to bite Belle, despite June telling it to go away. Belle was scared of dogs to a certain degree after her encounter with the ferocious animal.

Alvertie and her husband, Dallas Taylor, visited Etta as often as they could. Alvertie had always felt very close to her older sister. Dallas brought Belle a little red toothbrush with bristles attached to it. It was the first real toothbrush she had ever owned. June would get Belle's head in her lap and scrub her teeth with a cloth and soda to clean them in the past, but now Belle could clean her teeth extra well by herself. She was so proud of her little red toothbrush; she brushed her teeth every chance she had.

Despite Belle's regular brushing, she developed a cavity in one of her molars. Harrison took Belle to see Dr.

Mullins, a dentist in Newport, to have the tooth filled. Belle was terrified. Never having visited a dentist office until now, she did not know what to expect. Dr. Mullins told Belle to have a seat in the chair. This was the strangest chair she had ever seen. It had all kinds of unusual instruments surrounding it, and the big, bright light hurt her eyes. The doctor looked inside Belle's mouth and mumbled something under his breath. Without deadening the tooth, Dr. Mullins started grinding on the cavity. Belle let out a loud shriek as she came out of the chair and ran out into the lobby where her daddy waited. Dr. Mullins came out behind her. He told Harrison, "Bring her back in here."

"No, I won't! She's nervous, and you hurt her," Harrison answered as he took Belle by the hand. Harrison led his frightened daughter outside and they walked over to Maloy's Funeral Home, where the taxi stand stood. Soon the two were on their way back to Del Rio.

Harrison's grandmother, Lou Clements, had cancer on her foot, which made it difficult for her to walk. She was no longer able to care for herself, so Etta offered to take her into her care, which she did. Grandma Clements had a walking stick which she tapped on the floor when she wanted attention. Belle was amused by her great-grandmother and the stories she told of her experiences in life. Etta took comfort in being able to help someone in need. She always put the needs of others above her own.

Christmas Eve was here again. Belle loved to sit by the window and watch the snowflakes fall ever so gracefully from the sky. Even though it was dark outside now, the snow-covered valley reflected a soft white glow which allowed Belle to watch in awe as the big, fluffy flakes continued to fall. She gazed, almost in a trance, at one individual fluffy flake, and watched as it came down, down, down, until it finally came to rest on the glistening snow-covered ground. She thought, "How wonderful it would feel to be a snowflake...floating so free through the air, and..." Just then Belle's thoughts were interrupted by Etta telling her to get ready for bed. Going to bed was hard for Belle because she was so full of excitement on Christmas Eve, but Belle did as her mother instructed, "After all, Santa won't come as long as I'm awake," Belle concluded in her thoughts. She snuggled under the covers and soon drifted off. Etta pulled a chair up to the single window in the front room and set a big box in it, which "Santa" loaded with presents, then Etta went to bed, also.

Morning came...Christmas was here at last! Belle sprang from her bed and ran over to the box. As she peeped inside the box, she saw a tiny doll, an orange, apple, some nuts, and a juice harp for her. It thrilled her half to death to get the juice harp. She almost drove the family crazy playing with it all the time. The rest of the children received nuts and fruits; they were too old to receive toys now.

The year 1937 arrived. Spring brought new life to the mountains and new hope for the people living there. People started getting out of their cabins and houses, where they had all but hibernated during the winter, and started visiting friends and relatives. Picnics by one's favorite fishing hole filled the banks along the creek on Saturdays. People were stirring about once more without the encumbrance of heavy winter clothing and the cold wind whistling past their faces. Everyone loved spring in the mountains, including Etta.

While Emily was living in Newport, she attended special functions at the Tannery School where the woman she lived with, Emma Jones, taught. Emma's husband, Fred, told Emily there was a man he wanted her to meet at a pie supper the school was having. His name was Richard Gray Jones; his friends called him Dick. Emily baked a chess pie to be auctioned off at the at the school supper along with other pies the other women brought. During the auction Dick bought Emily's pie and the two became acquainted while making small talk as they ate it. Dick was quite smitten with Emily. After that night Dick and Emily began dating on a regular basis.

In January 1939 Harrison and Etta packed up their belongings and moved their family to a four-room house in an area known as Ground Squirrel, just about a mile or so from where they had been living. Ground Squirrel occupied an area of land just at the foot of Round Mountain. From the single window on the side of the living room one could view the beautiful, bold, Round Mountain in all its splendor.

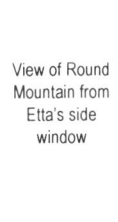

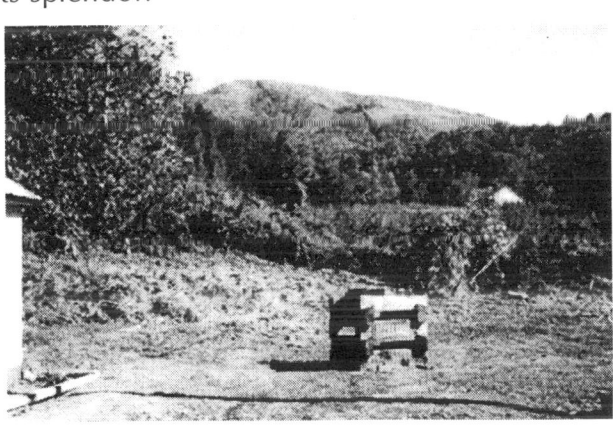

View of Round Mountain from Etta's side window

A bubbling little brook ran soothingly at the yard's edge in front of the house. A large front porch was made inviting by a porch swing and several wicker chairs. The kitchen held a woodstove and wooden cabinets on one end and was occupied by a large wooden eating table and a white cupboard on the other end. At the back of the kitchen wall was an entrance to a small bedroom; this would be Belle's room. At the back of the living room was an entrance to another bedroom. The living room contained a full-size bed on one side of the room, with a coal fireplace with several straightback chairs and small tables sitting nearby. Kerosene lamps set upon the tables, with Etta's homemade doilies adding a touch of cheerfulness to the room. Outside was a henhouse, smokehouse, a cellar for storing canned food and potatoes, a wash house, outside toilet, and a huge barn for milking and storage of hay and livestock food. On the other side of the brook, a dirt road led to wherever one might want to go. Across the road a steep, wooded bank offered some protection against the fierce westward winds which blew almost continuously during the month of March.

Harrison and Etta's closest neighbors were Jim and Ella Crowder, and above them lived Ishom Stinson in the house where Harrison and Etta were married. There was an empty house just below Harrison and Etta in the opposite direction down the road. This would be the last time Harrison and Etta would move; Harrison was buying this house and several acres of land surrounding it.

They had chosen a peaceful place with good neighbors. An air of contentment filled the house as it never had before in any of their previous homes. This house was, by far, a better house than the one they had lived in previously. Harrison would be 43 years old in October; Etta turned 42 on May 19th, Emily turned 22 on July 30th, June would be 20 on November 29th, Jack turned 16 on April 11th, and Belle turned 10 on May 2nd. The years were passing much too fast. Etta could not believe her firstborn child had already moved out to start a life of her own. June was hardly ever home anymore, and she feared Jack would soon be leaving, too. "Where has all the time gone?" Etta wondered to herself.

On August 5, 1939, Grandma Lou Clements passed away at the age of 90. Her frail, wrinkled body was placed in a casket in the back bedroom of Etta's house where family and friends could say their final good-bye. Friends brought food to Etta's house, and many of the neighbors stayed up all night with Harrison and Etta as they all mourned the passing of their loved one. The funeral service was held at the house the next day, then Grandma Clements was laid to rest in the Crowder Cemetery.

June was spending the weekend with Leora Willis and her husband, J. B., in Morristown when J. B. told June he wanted her to meet "T Boy," a good friend of his. T Boy's real name was John Thomas Gilliland. The arrangements were made for John to come by J. B.'s house on Sunday, which he did. John pulled up to J. B.'s house on Cumberland Street riding his motorcycle without the encumbrance of a helmet. June peered through the window to sneak a peek at her blind date as he dismounted his cycle. "Oh, he's the purttiest thang I've ever seen!" June whispered excitedly to a friend she had brought with her. It was love at first sight for both John and June. After their initial meeting, they began seeing one another steadily.

Etta's brother, Lurlie, took a bride on June 23rd earlier that same year. Iowa Willis became Mrs. Lurlie Grigsby, leaving J. L. the only child living at home with Novie. Lurlie and Iowa moved into the house Lurlie's grandfather, J. B. Grigsby, had lived in down in Slabtown.

On September 1, 1939, Hitler gave his German army the command to attack Poland. This would be the beginning of the most bloody war ever in history—World War II.

Months passed and with it came the happy union of Emily and Dick Jones as husband and wife on March 23, 1940. They made their first home a small house in the Irish Cut community, just North of Newport.

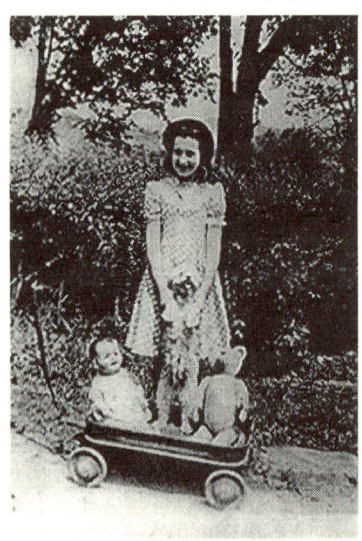

Belle Nichols, Age 11, holds her dog, Bootie, with her doll and teddy bear in wagon

At age 17 Jack joined the CCC (Civilian Conservation Corp.) in Bristol, Tennessee. They built bridges and did road work. The job paid $30 per month plus room and board. This was a lot of money for a young man, especially during the depression. Jack felt he had really hit it lucky. He headed out for Bristol with high hopes for the future. Now that Jack had left home, Belle was the only child Etta still had living with her. "Belle is only 11, so hopefully it will be awhile before I have to let go of my youngest child," Etta thought silently. It saddened her to watch her children leave home, one by one. She could not believe how fast they had grown up.

It was a warm day in April when Novie walked from her house in London up to Etta's for a visit. Novie stayed several hours helping Etta with small jobs around the house and chit-chatting about one thing or another. When Novie left the house to go home she was frightened by Belle, who was outside riding Jack's bicycle. Belle came down the dirt driveway straight toward Novie. She had her head down as if she was making her grandmother her target. As Belle sped closer, Novie threw up her hands and screamed, "Oh, Lordy!"

Belle stopped the bicycle just inches from her grandmother's legs. She never intended to hit her grandmother, but it scared Novie half to death. Etta came out on the porch when she heard her mother scream. Novie told Etta what Belle had done. Etta walked over to a nearby tree and broke off a limb. Belle's eyes widened as her mother approached her. Etta switched Belle on the legs several times with the hickory.

"I wasn't goin' ta run over her!" Belle cried.

"That don't matter. You scared her on purpose and that was wrong," Etta answered.

Belle walked off sobbing and heartbroken. This was the first time either of Belle's parents had used a hickory on her. As a matter of fact, Harrison had never spanked her at all; neither had Etta, but once or twice. This was a day Belle would never forget.

On September 2, 1940, 460,000 acres of the mountains, some on Tennessee land, and some on North Carolina land, was dedicated by President Franklin D. Roosevelt to become a part of the Great Smoky Mountains National Park. The people living in those parts of the mountains had to sell their land holdings to the U.S. Government. Only a few families remained in the area close to Max Patch. The black bear, white-tailed deer, bobcat, red fox, raccoon, wild boar, and wild turkey would now be free to thrive in the park.

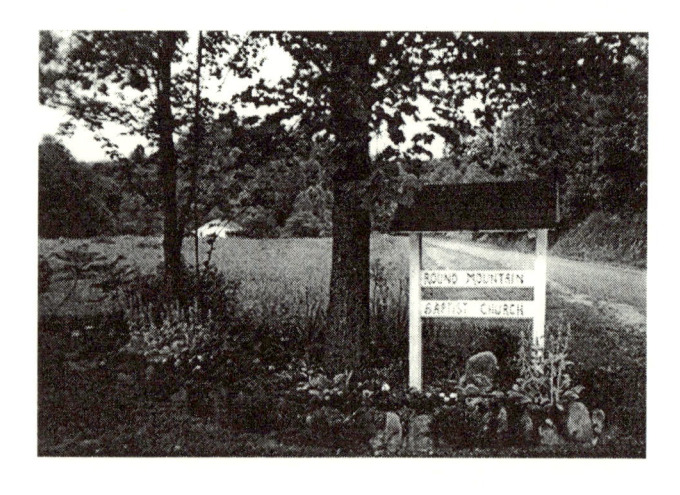

Round Mountain Church

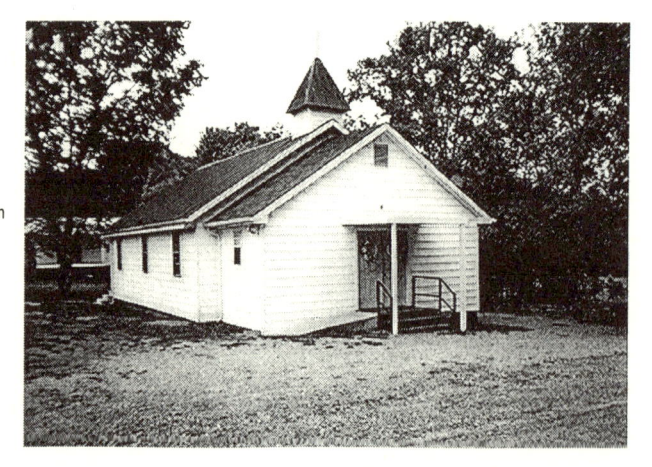

Etta "Granny" Nichols—Last of the Old-Timey Midwives

Harrison and Etta had been attending church at Round Mountain Church, located about one eighth of a mile from their house, ever since they moved to Ground Squirrel.

Etta made a point to invite the preacher and his family to come to her house for mid-day Sunday dinner every chance she could. On this particular Sunday, three preachers and their families had been invited to come to Etta's for dinner, but Etta was called away on a baby case. Harrison told the men to come anyway. "Belle can cook us some dinner," Harrison told them. Belle was only 13 years old. It made her so nervous to think she had to prepare a meal good enough for three preachers and their families. She went into the kitchen and opened a can of pickled green beans, fried some chicken, fried some potatoes, baked a pan of cornbread, and made a blackberry pie for dessert. Belle was pleased to see that everyone seemed to enjoy the meal she cooked, but she was upset with her father for some time, putting her in such an uncomfortable position.

In 1941 Jack quit working for the CCC in Bristol. The Depression was over, making work somewhat easier to obtain. He moved to Gastonia, North Carolina where he started working in the cotton mills. Later he returned to Tennessee and became an employee for TVA.

Etta took in her great aunt Laura Grigsby Greenwood to care for not long after Grandma Clements passed away. Laura was the sister to J. B. Grigsby. On June 20, 1941, Laura took her last breath around 8:30 P.M. on a Friday night. She was also placed in the back room, same as Grandma Clements, where friends could come to say their last good-bye. This service was also held at Harrison and

Etta's house. Aunt Laura was laid to rest in the Crowder Cemetery on South Highway 107 in the area known as Jonestown.

On December 7, 1941, Japan bombed Pearl Harbor around 7:55 A.M. The United States was now a fighting force involved in World War II. Many young men from Del Rio and surrounding communities were drafted into the Army to defend their country and preserve freedom. Mothers said good-bye to their sons, not knowing if they would ever see them alive again. Many recalled World War I, and knew neighbors or had relatives who were lost or injured in that war. Harrison's brother Claude had struggled with poor health ever since he returned home from serving in World War I because he had breathed too much of the poison gas used in battle. The people wondered how much devastation this war would bring to their country.

Part IV

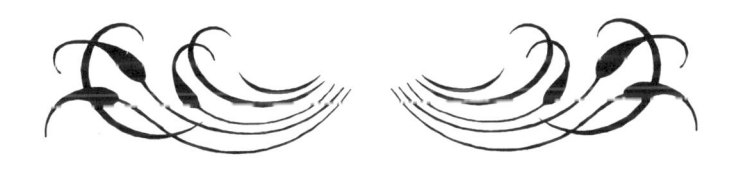

O Sweet Grandmother

Part IV

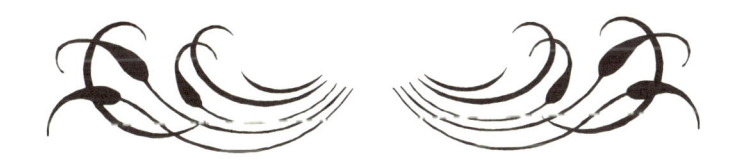

O Sweet Grandmother

John and June had been going steady ever since their first introduction. On August 16, 1941, John Thomas Gilliland took Bessie June Nichols as his bride. They were married by Rev. Brooks in his home in Morristown. June was 21 years old; John was 24. John was well liked by Harrison and Etta. They were happy to see their daughter marry such a good, upstanding young man. The happy couple settled in Morristown in a house on Montvue Avenue. June was very happy to get out of the mountains and vowed she would never go back to the hard life she experienced while growing up there.

More happy times came for Harrison and Etta when their first grandchild arrived on August 28th that same month. Etta was 49 years old when she became a grandmother for the first time. Etta took Carmel Seay's taxi to Dick and Emily's home in the Irish Cut a day or two before Emily went into labor. Emily gave birth to her first child as her mother performed the delivery. Oh, what a thrill this was for Etta when she took this little one in her arms after cutting the cord. "Its a girl, and she's just fine," Etta told Emily proudly. Etta cleaned the baby off and laid her in Emily's arms. The emotions were intense in the room as the proud mother and the proud grandmother both shared their excitement over the new little arrival. Dick came in after Etta had both mother and baby cleaned up and ready for him. He was a very proud father. Dick and Emily named their firstborn Valerie Jean Jones.

On May 12, 1942, June went into labor with her first baby. She was staying with her mother during the last days of her pregnancy so she would not have to rush from Morristown to get there on time. John was in the Army now; he would miss the birth of his first child. Dr. McGaha was June's doctor. Etta sent for him at the first signs of labor, but he was called away for emergency surgery in Greeneville this particular morning. Once again Etta was blessed with the privilege of delivering her grandchild. Etta checked June to see how far she was into labor. "The first one is always a little more stubborn 'bout comin' into the world. It'll be awhile yet," Etta reassured her daughter. "Don't try to rush it. Just let it happen," Etta continued.

Etta "Granny" Nichols—Last of the Old-Timey Midwives

Etta was never nervous about being a midwife, but when it was her own daughter giving birth it made her somewhat anxious until she knew for sure the baby and mother were both going to be okay. She did not let her daughter see her concern, though.

June grasped the iron bars on the headboard behind her tightly as the pains became more intense. "Oh, it hurts, Mama!" June screamed. Etta stood over her daughter and rubbed June's belly lightly when the bearing-down pains started. "Push! Its head is comin', June," Etta instructed.

June pushed with every ounce of strength she could muster. Her hands had the imprint of the design from the iron bars on them from squeezing the bars so tightly.

"One more time, June. It's a-comin'! It's a-comin'," Etta cried. With one final hard push, a beautiful dark-headed baby emerged into the world. "It's a girl, June, and she's so pretty!" Etta announced happily. Etta cleaned the baby up and put her in June's arms. "Now see if she'll drink some milk. Babies are usually hungry after getting born," Etta told June. June held the baby up to her breast and instinctively the cute little bundle of joy knew what to do. June decided on the name of Geraldine Ardys Gilliland for her new daughter.

As Etta walked into the living room to tell Harrison he had another granddaughter, a car pulled into Etta's driveway. It was Dr. McGaha. Harrison went out on the porch to greet the doctor and told him, "You're too late, Doc. She's already had the baby." After a bit of conversation, Dr. McGaha turned and walked back to his car and left. From there Dr. McGaha went down the road to check on Claude Nichols' mother-in-law. Belle happened to be there. Etta had sent her there when June started going into labor.

"Why, if you're 13 years old they should have let you stay," Dr. McGaha told Belle. "You're old enough to start learning about such stuff," he continued. Belle just smiled, being slightly embarrassed by his remark.

June stayed with her mother for several days after giving birth. She sent word to John in the Army that the baby had arrived. John arranged to get a pass to come home as soon as he got the news. When he walked into Etta's house, June was sitting in the rocker with the baby in her arms. John walked over to June and looked down in amazement at his child. At that moment Geraldine made a horrible face, probably caused from gas. "That's the ugliest baby I've ever seen!" John said jokingly. June got tickled, and the room was soon filled with laughter. It was good to have John home with his family for this special occasion. He would have to leave to return to the Army in just a few days.

On May 16, 1943, Jack entered the U.S. Navy during one of the worst wars ever recorded. With tears in her eyes, Etta said good-bye to her only son. Jack took a taxi to the Del Rio train depot. There he began his journey bound for Bane Bridge, Maryland, where he would undergo nine weeks of boot camp. After his basic training, Jack was ordered to serve on the U.S.S. Intrepid CVII battleship, which was stationed at the Marshall Islands. From there the ship would go on to Japan. Etta had to place all her faith in God to watch over Jack and bring him back home safe.

Etta "Granny" Nichols—Last of the Old-Timey Midwives

Not only did Etta have to worry about her only son going to war, she also had the worry of her two younger brothers who were already in the service. Furman was drafted into the Army in 1941. Furman received his basic training in Springfield, Louisiana. There he met Mary Maggio. After a brief courtship they were married before Furman was ordered to leave the country to go to Italy. Furman and Mary planned to settle in Baton Rouge, Louisiana, upon Furman's return from the Army.

J. L. was drafted into the Army in 1942. He received his basic training at St. Louis, Missouri. J. L. and Holland Greene were the only two men from Del Rio who did not get to come home on leave before being shipped off overseas. J. L. was ordered to leave

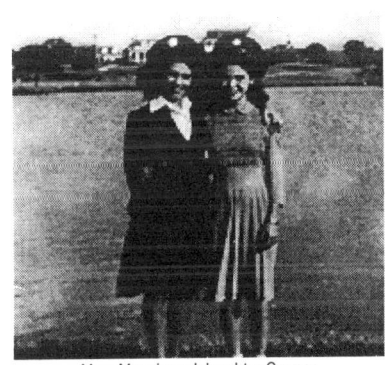

Mary Maggio and daughter Carman

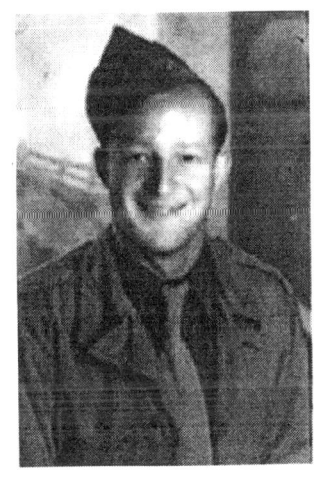

Furman Grigsby

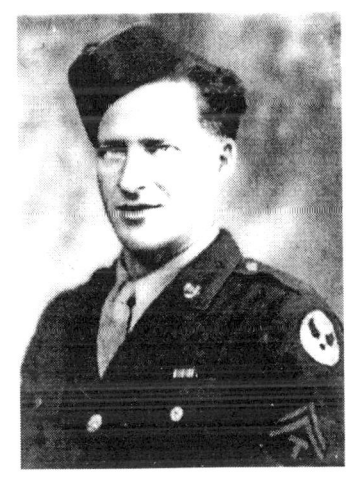

J. L. Grigsby

immediately after finishing his basic training and go to England. J. L. would spend the next four years and two months fighting in battle all through Europe before he would get to come home.

On November 24, 1943, Etta stood beside Emily's bed at her home in Irish Cut as she gave birth to her second baby. Doctor McGaha came to perform the delivery. Emily squeezed her mother's hand as her final push brought a tiny baby girl into the world. She was named Barbara Dean Jones. Etta looked at Dr. McGaha with an expression of a very concerned grandmother. She knew something was wrong with the baby. Her color was not normal. She was a "blue baby." Dr. McGaha confirmed what Etta feared: Barbara Dean had an enlarged heart. Etta knew her tiny little grandbaby would not survive.

Several days later, two year old Valerie watched as her grandmother sat in the wooden rocking chair crying as she gently rocked her granddaughter in her arms. Barbara Dean was dying and there was nothing Etta or the doctors could do, but Etta could make sure her granddaughter knew how much she was loved. After a brief life of six days, Barbara Dean died on November 30th. She was buried at Union Cemetery in Newport.

The year 1944 arrived. Jack had been interested in a beautiful young woman by the name of Juanita Finchum for some time. He first met her when he went to school at Mulberry Gap. He used to save her a seat on the school bus when the family lived at Blue Mill. Jack always spent as much time as he could with Juanita on his home passes from the Navy. Things were looking pretty serious in the romance department for these two.

Etta "Granny" Nichols—Last of the Old-Timey Midwives

Belle had been courting for a couple of years now, too. Belle had a close friend, Eulalah Seay, who worked in her father's store in Slabtown. One day, Floyd J. Smith came into the store when Eulalah was there. He was home on a pass from the Army. Floyd and Furman were both drafted into the Army around the same time. Floyd was the third son of Art Smith and Mary Caroline Bible Smith, the midwife who had delivered Etta's first child.

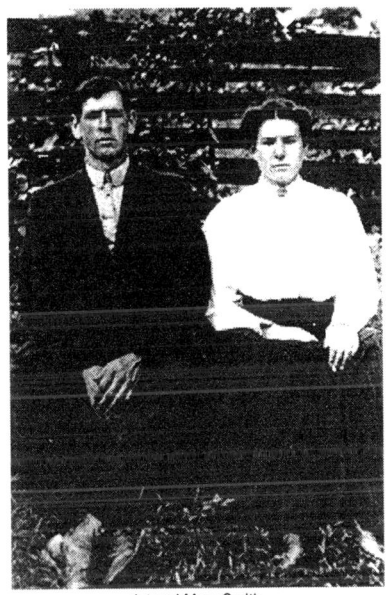

Art and Mary Smith

Eulalah showed Floyd a picture of Belle while he was in the store. Floyd's interest in the pretty redhead was immediate. He wrote Belle a letter from Fort Knox, Kentucky, where he was stationed at that time, telling her how he saw her picture and he would like to meet her. After that, Belle and Floyd started corresponding by mail on a regular basis. On Floyd's next pass home, he

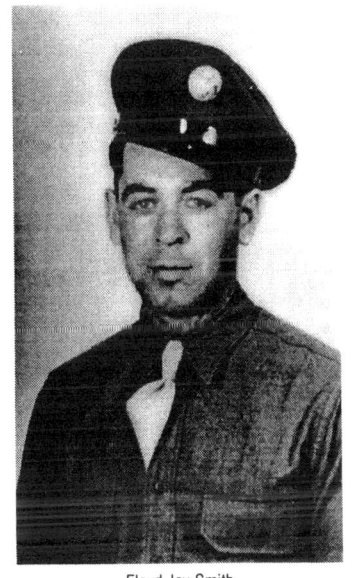

Floyd Jay Smith

finally got to meet Belle in person. The two hit it off from the start.

Belle remembered her Uncle Furman telling a story about when he and Floyd went to a holiness church to play music together. They used to travel all over the countryside making music at different churches and social gatherings. Furman said, "At this particular church, the people was a-shoutin' all over there, and they'd dance around and knock us down. Floyd was bad to get tickled, and I thought he would laugh out right there, but he didn't. They'uz dancin' I mean all over that church. This woman was slingin' her arms and skipping from one side of that church to the other. Floyd looked at me and said, 'Do you know what you're playin' now?' And I said, 'Yeah, but just keep it up. They don't know no better.' Now we wasn't singin' it, so they didn't know what we'uz playin'. We'uz playin' *Goin' Down the Road Feelin' Bad, Ain't Gonna Be Treated This A'way*. And I just kept a goin', and I bet we played that song for 30 minutes. So when we finally quit, we got outta there, and I thought Floyd would die a-laughin', cause when he got tickled, he got tickled!"

During another pass home from the Army, Floyd and Belle made plans to elope the following morning. It was a crisp, cool, fall morning when Belle was awakened by the crowing of the rooster. This was her wedding day. She got dressed quickly and rushed out the front door. While Harrison and Etta were at the barn milking the cow, Belle ran down the road to meet Floyd who was waiting for her in a car. They rode to Greenville, South Carolina where they were married by the Honorable Guy Gullick.

When Harrison and Etta returned from the barn, Harrison stepped into the kitchen from the back door and saw the kitchen still in a mess from the morning meal. He turned to Etta and said, "I just want you to look, Doc. Baby Girl left without even cleaning up the kitchen!" This was not like Belle. Harrison did not know what to make of it.

As soon as Floyd and Belle said their vows, they headed back for Tennessee. When arriving in Del Rio, they went to Floyd's parents house in Slabtown, where they stayed for the night. The next morning they went to see Harrison and Etta. Floyd was afraid of how Harrison might react at the news of their marriage. He walked slowly up the steps on the side of the front porch, dreading what he had to do next. Floyd and Belle explained to Harrison and Etta about where they had been and how they were now married. Belle's parents were shocked by the news, but remained as calm as they possibly could under the circumstances. It was decided that Belle would remain living with her parents until Floyd was discharged from the Army. Floyd returned to Fort Knox, Kentucky, the next day, leaving Belle in the capable hands of her parents.

Later that same year, on December 30, 1944, Jack and Juanita were married by Rev. J. J. Johnson in Newport. Jack was in on a home pass from the Navy. The two newlyweds spent the night at Harrison and Etta's. Juanita would live with her parents until Jack was discharged from the Navy. Juanita's parents house was located about one

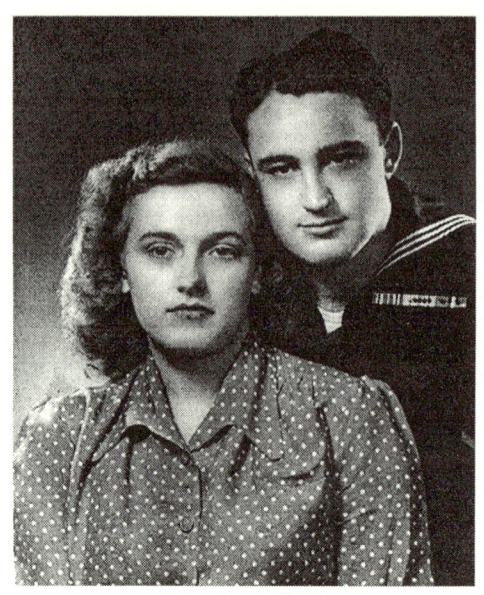

Jack and Juanita Nichols

mile away from Harrison and Etta's house, down in a peaceful valley just off South Highway 107.

Floyd received orders to go to France in February of 1945. This was very upsetting news for Floyd and Belle because Belle was pregnant with their first child. The baby was due sometime in late June or early July of that year. Floyd received a pass to come home for several days before having to ship out for France. Floyd said his goodbyes to his family and his wife, not knowing how long it would be before he would see them again.

It was a warm morning on June 10, 1945, when Etta returned from milking the cow. She poured the fresh milk from the bucket into the milk crocks, just as she had done every morning for as long as she could remember. Just then she heard a truck pull up in her driveway. It was Claude Stokely. Claude's long slender legs carried him to

Etta "Granny" Nichols—Last of the Old-Timey Midwives

the front door in fast strides. He pounded on the door with his fist so hard it almost made Etta drop the milk bucket.

"Etter, can you come to my house? Bonnie has been painin' quite fierce this mornin'. I thank it's time fer the baby to come," Claude pleaded anxiously.

"Why, sure I can. Let me cover my milk and get my medical bag, and I'll be ready to go." Etta walked to the edge of the porch and hollered to Harrison, who was working in the fields, telling him she was going on a "baby case." Harrison acknowledged her with a wave good-bye, then Etta climbed into the pickup truck with Claude. Claude and Bonnie lived in Spice Wood Flats, several miles away. When Etta arrived at their house, she checked Bonnie and timed her pains. This was Claude and Bonnie's first baby, so Etta knew patience would have to be practiced on her part. Noon came and the baby still had not come. Claude's mother was there to help do whatever she could. She prepared the noon meal for the others. Etta helped with the dishes afterwards. Time passed. It was after 6 P.M. when Bonnie started having hard labor pains.

"She's havin' harder miseries now. It won't be much longer," Etta told Mrs. Stokely, who was standing beside Bonnie's bed.

Bonnie squeezed Mrs. Stokely's hand as the pains grew stronger and stronger. At 7 P.M., Bonnie gave birth to a 10 1/2-pound baby girl. Etta cleaned the baby off and put her in Bonnie's arms.

"Have you decided what you're gonna name 'er? I need to put it on the birth certificate," Etta said.

"Yeah, we've decided to name 'er Dora Kate Stokely," Bonnie answered.

Mother and baby were both fine, so Etta went into the kitchen and fixed the family some supper before asking Claude to take her home.

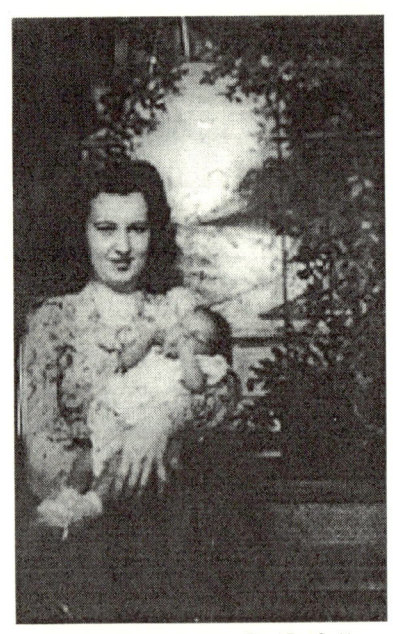

On Saturday, June 30, 1945, Belle began having labor pains. On Sunday morning Etta sent for Dr. McGaha, Belle's doctor. He arrived Sunday afternoon. It was getting late in the evening so Dr. McGaha stayed all night at Etta's while waiting on the new arrival. Monday morning came. It was a hot day on July 2nd when Belle's water finally broke. Around 11:15 A.M. Dr. McGaha put Belle to sleep—he was going to have to use forceps to help get the baby out. At 11:30 a big nine-pound baby boy entered the world. He had dark hair and brown eyes. It was some time before Belle woke up. She opened her eyes to find her new son in her arms and her mother lying on the bed beside her getting some rest. The baby was named Floyd Ray Smith. When Belle felt up to it she wrote Floyd a letter telling him about the birth of his son. It was a shame Floyd could not be there for the birth of his first child.

Belle holds her newborn son, Floyd Ray Smith

On September 2, 1945, the announcement America had been waiting to hear for six long years finally came: World War II was over! Victory celebrations broke out all across the country as the details came across the radio of how the atomic bomb was dropped on Hiroshima, Japan, causing the enemy to surrender.

On November 28, 1945, Floyd received his honorable discharge from the U.S. Army. He served in the 417th Ordnance Evacuation Company. He brought home the American Theater Ribbon, World War II Victory Medal, European African Middle Eastern Ribbon, and a Good Conduct Medal.

Floyd's reunion with his family was a happy one. He finally held his new baby boy for the first time when Floyd Ray was four months old. A proud, wide smile overtook Floyd's expression as Belle handed him his firstborn child. He was a big boy for his age. Floyd said, "That's because he comes from good, healthy stock."

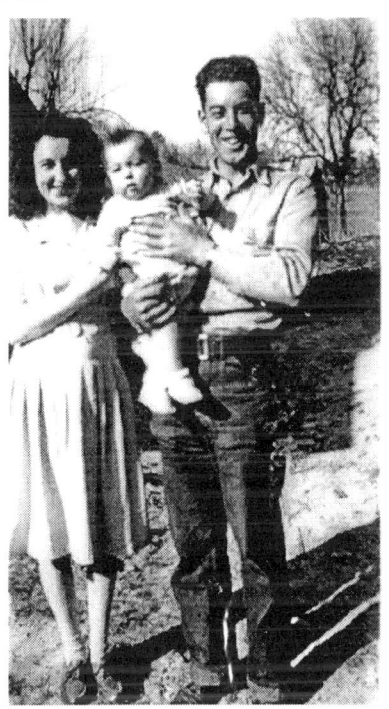

Floyd and Belle Smith with their baby, Floyd Ray in 1946

Art and Mary Smith, Floyd's parents, bought a large tract of land just above Slabtown soon after Floyd returned from the Army. It had an attractive little white house located on it where Art and Mary were living. They hoped their ten children would choose to build their homes on some of the property. Mary's most cherished wish was to keep her children close to her. Over time, Mary would see her wish come true and the tract of land she and Art bought would come to be known as Smithville.

Art and Mary discussed selling some of the land to Floyd and Belle as a place to build their first home. Floyd accepted the offer. He was a good carpenter, as were his brothers, so it would not take long to get the house finished with their help. Floyd and Belle picked out an area at the upper end of the property, and the construction of the house soon began.

On January 19, 1946, J. L. Grigsby married Loiree Smith. She was the daughter of Art and Mary Smith, the younger sister of Floyd. Loiree was 23 years old and J. L. was 28. They picked out a plot of land in Smithville towards the middle of the tract on which they would build their house.

Novie was living alone now that J. L. was married, but she had already grown accustomed to it ever since J. L. had left for the Army. She moved into a small house in Slabtown on the side of the road just past the turnoff onto Midway road.

In March of 1946, Floyd and Belle moved into their new house in Smithville. Etta sure would miss having her baby grandson living there with her. She had helped bathe, feed, and care for him ever since he was born. It was like she was having to let go of one of her own children.

It was a cool morning in April 1946 when a knock came at Etta's door. A young woman stood on the porch holding a baby in her arms. Etta opened the door and invited her in.

I'm here to see if you will take my baby and raise him," replied the woman. "I just ain't able to feed 'im anymore and take care of 'im the way he needs. Some of my friends told me 'bout you and how much you love babies, so I thought you'd be able to give 'im a good home."

Etta's eyes lighted up with excitement as she answered, "Well, of course I'll take 'im. What's his name?"

"His name is Joy, and he'll be nine months old in two more weeks."

"Why, he's just about the same age as my grandson, Floyd Ray. You just leave Joy with me and don't worry 'bout 'im. He'll be well took care of."

The lady gave Etta the few belongings she had for her son then hugged him tight. She put Joy in Etta's arms and turned to leave. She gave one last glance at the baby she had to leave behind as she walked out the door, tears streaming down her cheeks. The car she came in backed out of Etta's driveway, and she was gone.

Etta could hardly believe God had blessed her in this way. She could not wait to tell Harrison. She hoped he would come home soon. When Harrison finally did come home from the fields he found Etta sitting in her wooden rocking chair rocking the baby. At first he thought it was Floyd Ray, then he realized it was not. Etta began telling Harrison about the single mother who brought the baby to them to raise, and how she had accepted the woman's offer. "What! Doc, have you taken leave of your senses?! We can't take on raisin' another young'un at our age!

You'll have to find someone else to take the baby," Harrison declared firmly.

"I'll do no such a thing," Etta snapped back. "We can raise this baby just as good as anybody else 'round here. Besides, you won't have to take care of 'im. I'll be the one doin' most of the work. I want to keep 'im...and I'm gonna keep 'im!" Etta's face was blood red with anger towards Harrison. "Does he not know how much I want another child? All of my children are gone, and I need another child to feel complete again," Etta thought to herself. The two argued for several days over the situation concerning the baby. Harrison would not back down from his decision; neither would Etta. On the third day Etta came out of her bedroom with a sack of clothes in one arm and Joy in the other. She told Harrison she was leaving him if he would not agree to let her keep the child. Harrison still did not budge from his decision. Etta walked out the door and started down the road. The April air was cool and light. Etta had on a heavy winter coat and had the baby bundled up tight under a heavy homemade baby quilt. She walked a little over one mile carrying Joy and the paper sack full of clothes before she came to Belle and Floyd's house. Etta walked up the steps on the front porch and knocked on the door. Belle was surprised to find her mother standing at the door with a bag of clothes and...a baby? She invited her mother to come inside as she took the sack from Etta's arms to lighten her mother's load. "What in the world is going on, Mother? Whose baby is that?" Belle asked curiously.

Etta told Belle the story of how she acquired the baby. "Your dad is just too stubborn for his own good! I'm leavin' 'im. Let 'im see how hard it is to get by when I'm not there to do for 'im." cried Etta.

"Why, Mother, you know Daddy can't cook. What'll he eat? Why, he'll starve to death with you gone."

"I don't care. He don't worry 'bout what I want, so why should I worry 'bout him? I just want to know if I can stay with you fer awhile 'til I decide what I'm gonna do," Etta asked in a quavering voice.

"Well, of course you can stay here. Bring your things in here to the bedroom," Belle said as she led her mother through the hallway. "You can sleep in here with the baby."

Nightfall came. Belle and Etta lit the oil lamps and cleared the supper dishes from the table. "Mother, you go watch Floyd Ray and Joy, and I'll wash the dishes," Belle instructed her mother. After the dishes were done and the kitchen wiped clean, Belle joined her mother and Floyd in the living room. Etta had both the boys ready for bed. Floyd Ray was placed in his crib in Floyd and Belle's bedroom. Joy was put to bed in the room where Etta would sleep. Etta placed pillows in front of Joy to prevent him from rolling out onto the floor. Etta returned to the living room and picked up The Holy Bible which lay on Belle's coffee table. She always read a chapter every night before going to bed. Tonight she was extremely restless. Being upset with Harrison had sapped her energy, but being in a strange place, and wondering what she should do, made it hard to fall asleep. Most of Etta's night was spent tossing and turning in bed. She woke up every hour or so to check on Joy. He was restless, too, being surrounded by strangers.

Morning arrived, after what seemed to Etta to be one of the longest nights she had experienced in awhile. Floyd arose early to go out on his job with Arthur E. Smith, his brother-in-law. They worked in the lumber business together. Belle always got up when Floyd did to prepare breakfast. After the morning dishes were washed, Belle took Floyd Ray and Joy in front of the wood stove in the living room and gave them both their morning bath. Etta helped Belle with the housework and the babies.

Three days passed. Harrison had not made any attempt to persuade his wife to come home. Belle was feeling sorry for her daddy because she knew how helpless he was in the kitchen. She understood how both her parents felt about raising another baby. It made it terribly difficult for her to voice her opinion on the subject with her mother.

Etta finally realized, without any outside influence from her daughter, she had no choice but to find another home for Joy. She knew that Charlie and Eunice Barrett had been trying to have a baby unsuccessfully for some time. She would approach them first to see if they wanted Joy to raise as their own. The couple was delighted to take the baby. Etta returned home to Harrison. They made up with one another, but Etta's heart ached from having to give up the baby. She would hold some resentment towards Harrison for a long time to come.

Several months later, the young woman who had brought Joy to Etta returned to her doorway. She was there to get her baby back. "The father of my baby is with me now, and with his help I'll be able to raise Joy," the lady said joyfully.

"Well, I'm afraid I don't have Joy here anymore. Harrison, my husband, wouldn't let me keep 'im. So I found a real nice couple that wanted to take him in," Etta informed her. Etta told the woman how to get to the house where her son was now living. The woman thanked Etta for helping her son then turned and left.

Etta went to visit Charlie and Eunice later. They had to let the baby go with his birth mother. They were both brokenhearted that their chance of raising a child had been taken away. (God would later bless this kind, good-hearted couple with eight children of their own.)

On June 19, 1946, Claude Stokely made another trip to Etta's house to fetch her. His wife, Bonnie, was in labor with their second child. It was around noon when Etta walked into the Stokely home. The air was hot, with the first day of summer just around the corner. Etta wiped the sweat from her face with a handkerchief she had taken from Harrison's bureau drawer as she walked into the bedroom where Bonnie would give birth. After the usual questions, Etta washed her hands with soap and rinsed them in the hottest water she could stand. She then checked Bonnie to see how far along she was in labor. "It'll be a couple of hours yet," Etta told Bonnie. Etta sat down in a straightback chair beside Bonnie's bed. She took a cool, wet rag and placed it on Bonnie's forehead. It was miserably hot inside the house. Etta stayed at Bonnie's side waiting for the little one to arrive. Bonnie's sister, Dussie Norwood, kept Dora Kate in the front room while her mother was giving birth. At 4 P.M. Bonnie gave birth to an 8 1/2-pound baby boy. Claude and Bonnie were both thrilled. They named him James Joseph Stokely.

Fall of 1946 arrived cooling the hot, humid air which made life so uncomfortable. Etta often kept Floyd Ray with her at her house. One morning as Etta stood at the kitchen sink washing dishes, Floyd Ray, who was cutting teeth, toddled up behind her and bit her on the hip. Etta, as an instant reflex, swung her hand around and accidentally hit Floyd Ray in the face. Floyd Ray began squalling at the top of his lungs as he turned and walked back into the living room. Etta followed trying to console him and making sure he was not physically hurt from her slap. The biggest hurt was Floyd Ray's pride. His grandmother had never done such a thing to him before. He just could not understand why she slapped him, but his crying sure did seem to get his grandmother's attention, so he was not about to stop. "He cried and cried. I didn't think I was ever goin' to get 'im to hush. You know I wouldn't hurt any young'un on purpose. I believe it hurt me more'n it did him." Etta told Belle later that day.

"Well, he's probably already forgotten about it, Mother. Don't blame yourself. You just reacted the same as anybody else would have," Belle reassured her mother.

Etta put some iodine on her bite and never mentioned it in front of Floyd Ray again.

On September 24, 1946, Earnest Wilburn rode to Etta's house on his horse. He came to take Etta to his house in Midway. His wife, Eula Mae, whom everyone called Kate, was ready to give birth to their sixth child. Etta grabbed her coat and medical bag, then mounted the horse with Earnest. The air was colder than usual for this time of the year. There had already been a frost which killed a lot of peoples' tobacco crops, including Earnest's.

Etta had delivered all but one of Earnest and Kate's children in the past years. She delivered Kenneth Robert on March 15, 1940; Bertie Marie, who was named after Marie Smith, on December 15, 1941; John David on September 19, 1943; Earnest Troy on October 7, 1945; and now she was back again. Mary Bible Smith delivered their first child, James Perry, on September 20, 1938. Etta was there for five to six hours before Kate gave birth to a little girl. They named her Mary Frances. Etta stayed another hour after the birth to make sure mother and baby were okay. She collected a fee of $5 then Earnest gave her a ride back to her house on his horse. Earnest and Kate thought a lot of Etta. Kate appreciated the way Etta took care of her each time she delivered a baby. Sometimes Etta cooked a meal for the family while she was there, if there was no one to help out. She had a kind spirit that touched everyone in a special way.

It was a cold day on February 1, 1947, when June went into labor with her second child. Dr. McGaha was sent for in Newport to come to June's home in Morristown to perform the delivery. Etta could not be there this time due to bad weather and the distance of the journey. June gave birth to another baby girl. She was named Virginia Ann Gilliland. Etta now had four living grandchildren at the age of 49.

J. L. and Loiree became the proud parents of their first child on March 30, 1947. They had a baby girl which they named Deloris Dianne Grigsby. The delivery was performed by Dr. Nease at J. L. and Loiree's home. The baby weighed 8 1/4-pounds.

Six months later, Jack and Juanita became the proud parents of Susan Loye Nichols. She was born on October 29, 1947, at Jack and Juanita's home they rented from Tilman Ball in Del Rio. Dr. McGaha and Dr. Shults performed the delivery of the 9-pound baby girl with fair skin, pretty blond hair, and blue eyes.

On March 30, 1948, Belle went into labor with her second baby. Floyd drove her up to Etta's. Dr. McGaha was sent for in Newport, also. Belle was only eight months into her pregnancy. Etta told Belle to lie down in the bed in the bedroom next to the living room. When Dr. McGaha arrived he checked Belle. He took Etta over to one side of the room. "The baby isn't trying to help itself. It isn't moving at all," Dr. McGaha said. Etta looked worried as she walked over to Belle. Dr. McGaha told Belle of his suspicion about the baby. "You will have to do all the work to get this baby born, Belle," he said. Belle pushed with all her strength. Dr. McGaha finally got a grip on the baby and helped pull it out. He was right—the baby was dead. "I think it has probably been dead about two weeks," he told Belle in a dismal tone. Etta took the baby and wrapped it in a blanket. She placed the baby on the cedar chest next to the wall. Belle never saw her stillborn son.

The next morning Floyd went to Newport to buy a casket for his son. Several of Belle's aunts came to offer their help the same morning. Wylie Sexton came down, also. He told Etta, "I didn't know what was wrong. I just had a real strong feelin' that I needed to come down here, and here I am." Wylie helped Harrison dig a grave for his stillborn grandson on the hill next to Harrison and Etta's house. The baby was placed in the casket Floyd brought back, and he was buried on the hill. Floyd and Belle wanted to give their child a name regardless of the unfortunate circumstances. He was named Gary Smith.

In the summer of 1948 electricity came to Del Rio. Bob Raines wired most of the houses in the community to receive this miracle flow of energy. No longer did Etta have to heat her clothes iron on the stove; the oil lamps could be put away, and electrical appliances for the home could make life a little easier.

One of the first electrical appliances Etta bought was an electric churn. This was the best thing to come into Etta's life since buttermilk! No longer did she have to stand for hours churning the milk by hand to make butter. She just plugged up her new electric churn, and it did the work for her, allowing her more time to spend on other chores. Etta told all her family and friends about her new churn and advised them to buy one as soon as they could.

Floyd and Belle were the first family in the community to buy an electric refrigerator. It was a Sears Cold Spot. The man Floyd bought it from got in touch with Floyd a few days later and told him he had three more if he knew of anyone else wanting to buy one. Floyd's parents bought one; his sister, Iva Freeman and her husband, Boyd, bought one; and J. L. and Loiree bought one. All these families lived in Smithville and were considered to be "well off" by some of the other families in the community. Jealousy spread around the area as word got out about the refrigerators. People talked about Floyd having the first inside bathroom in his house, also. They figured Floyd was biting off more than he could chew financially, but Floyd never did have to let anything go back. He was a hard worker and he paid for everything through long hours of labor and sweat, as did all the families living in Smithville.

Etta continued to go on baby cases. On October 12, 1948, Claude Stokely pulled into Etta's driveway. She was off to deliver his and Bonnie's third baby. It was mid-afternoon when Etta arrived at their home in Spicewood Flats. The weather was unseasonably cold for early October.

"You know, it feels like it might just come a good snow," Etta told Bonnie, trying to take her mind off the labor pains. She continued making small talk until Bonnie's "miseries" got stronger. At 9 P.M. Bonnie gave birth to a 9-pound baby girl. They named her Nellie Mae Stokely.

Etta was right about the snow. It started pouring down just before Nellie was born. Etta rushed to get her things together so Claude could take her home before the roads became impassable. "Everything looks to be just fine with Bonnie and the baby, or I'd stay longer," Etta told Claude. He was just as anxious as Etta to get her home and get back home himself, before the ground became covered with snow. Etta collected $5 for her services then returned home.

The next year brought happier times back into Etta and her children's lives. On June 20, 1949, Emily gave birth to a healthy baby girl. Dick and Emily named their precious bundle, Sandra Kay Jones. Etta helped Dr. McGaha perform the delivery.

Several months later, on October 9, 1949, Belle went into labor with her third child. It was late afternoon when

Belle had her first pain. Floyd drove her up to her mother's house then he drove on to Newport to get Dr. McGaha. Floyd Ray stayed with Floyd so he would not get in the way at Etta's house. Harrison's mother, Martha Crowder, happened to be there when Floyd dropped Belle off. She stood beside Belle's bed as Etta heated a pan of hot water on the wood cookstove. She took the hot water in the bedroom and set it down on a stool beside the bed. Just then Belle's water broke. Etta turned to quickly wash her hands.

"Etter, it's a-comin'! It's a-comin', Etter!" Martha said excitedly as she held Belle's knees. This baby was in a hurry to stretch its legs.

Etta got there just in time to catch the baby. It was a baby girl this time. She weighed 9-pounds, same as her older brother, Floyd Ray. She had black curly hair and blue eyes. Belle and Floyd had chosen the name Linda Carol Smith for a girl.

Floyd arrived shortly after Linda was born. "The doctor was gone on another case," Floyd said as he came through the front door.

Etta giggled, "Well, it don't matter now. Belle's done had the baby."

Floyd quickly walked into the bedroom where he met his beautiful little baby girl lying in her mother's arms. Floyd Ray came in next to meet his baby sister. He stood in wondering reverence as he peered at the wrinkled, squirmy little thing they called his sister. He asked his mother, "Where did she come from? She wasn't here when we left awhile ago."

"We'll tell you 'bout it when you're a little older," Floyd laughed.

Etta took Floyd Ray by the hand and led him out of the room. Belle stayed with her mother for two or three days while she regained her strength before returning to her home.

Emily, Valerie, and Sandra usually caught Carmel Seay's taxi on Saturday afternoon from their home in Irish Cut to go to Harrison and Etta's. Carmel charged a fee of 25 cents for the 20 mile journey. Emily and the children stayed all night at her parents' home so they could go to church at Round Mountain Church the following day. Etta and Harrison enjoyed having their daughter and grandchildren visit with them on the weekends. Dick would come up late on Sunday evening to drive his wife and children back home.

On this particular Sunday, seven-year-old Valerie saw her father pulling into the driveway at Etta's. She rushed out to the porch to greet him. Dick could see something curled up on the steps on the side of the porch as he came up the driveway. It was dusk, which prevented him from being able to make out what the curled object was until he got closer. Then he saw it—a large yellow-and-black diamondback rattlesnake! Valerie was starting down the steps! Dick sped up the driveway to the steps, jumped out of the car, and grabbed Valerie just before she was about to step on the deadly reptile. The snake crawled off the step and went under the house. Dick took Valerie inside. Shaken, Dick told Harrison and the others about the snake.

"Well, I'll have to find it and kill it or it might bite someone else, then I'd feel like I was to blame 'cause I didn't kill it when I had the chance," Harrison said.

Harrison went to the bedroom and got his gun and a lantern. He went outside and crawled under the porch. He searched cautiously through the rubble and dirt, having only the light from the lantern to see by, since it was now dark outside. Harrison heard a noise just ahead in some old baskets he had stored under the house. He picked up a rock from the ground and threw it at the baskets. The rattle of the snake's buttons became very loud. There it was! He could see it now. Harrison aimed his gun and quickly squeezed the trigger...BANG! He got it! The snake was dead. Harrison had taken quite a risk going under the house in the dark to kill a rattlesnake. It could very easily have bitten him before he realized he was upon it, but God had surely been with him, protecting him from the deadly venomous creature. Harrison crawled out from under the porch with the dead snake in his hand. Etta and the rest of the family were standing on the porch. Harrison held the snake up to show the others.

"This was an old feller. He has 16 buttons on his rattler, and just look how big he is!" Harrison said as he held up his trophy.

"I want you to know!" Etta said in a tone of disbelief as she gazed at the large snake.

"I tell you what! I've never moved so fast in my life as I did when I saw Valerie fixin' to step on that thing!" Dick said as he wiped his forehead with his sleeve.

"I'm glad to know you got it, Daddy, instead of it gettin' you," Emily said with a sigh of relief.

After the excitement was over. Dick and Emily gathered the girls and started back to their house. Valerie would never forget the horrifying experience she had gone through this night.

On April 9, 1950, Jack took Juanita to Valentine-Shults Hospital in Newport where they became the proud parents of an 11-pound baby boy. Dr. McGaha and Dr. Shults performed the delivery. Jack and Juanita named their son James Lewis Nichols; they would call him Jimmy.

On September 9, 1950, June gave birth to a son at her home in Morristown. Etta was present to assist in the delivery. Dr. McGaha was also present to perform the delivery. John and June named their baby boy Thomas James Gilliland; he would go by the name of Tommy. Tommy had a heart defect at birth. Dr. McGaha did not know how long Tommy could live, but it did not look very promising for Tommy to live a long life. Of course, this was very upsetting for John and June, and Etta as well. Etta had already seen her other two daughters go through the heartache of losing a baby; now it appeared June would experience it, also. Etta's heart went out to her daughter, and especially to her tiny, defenseless grandson. Once again Etta was overwhelmed by her feeling of helplessness. At times like this Etta had to trust that God had a good reason for allowing such things to happen to her family. She had to trust in Him to give her and her family the strength to get through the hard times...and He always did.

It was a crisp, chilly day on November 9, 1950, when Charles Love Cagle came to Etta's house to take her to his home on Bull Mountain. Love's wife, Oree, was in labor.

Etta helped assist in the delivery of the Cagle's first child when they lived on Baker's Branch three years previously. Dr. Walter Smith was there, also, to perform the delivery. Oree gave birth to an 8-pound baby boy that time. They named him Harold Cagle. He was born on April 22, 1947, around 10 A.M.

Etta and Love reminisced about Harold's birth as he drove her up the winding dirt road to his house. It was 10 A.M. when Love and Etta reached his home. Oree was lying in her bed. Etta went through her usual routine, which she performed on all her patients about to give birth. It was around noon when Oree gave birth to an 8-pound baby girl. Oree and Love named their little beauty Irene Phyllis Cagle. Oree and Love paid Etta $10 for her services. Etta stayed another two hours after the birth before Love took her home.

J. L. and Loiree Grigsby celebrated the birth of a new son on November 16, 1950. Loiree's youngest brother, Arthur, went to Newport to pick up Dr. Nease to perform the delivery. At 9:00 A.M. Thursday morning Loiree gave birth to a 9-pound baby boy at her home in Smithville. They named him Michael Arthur Grigsby.

Spring of 1951 arrived bringing bright sunshine and warmer temperatures. Floyd Ray was staying with Etta one day when he decided to go out in the backyard and practice throwing Etta's butcher knife. Of course, Etta did not see Floyd Ray get the knife; she never would have allowed him to play with it. Five-year-old Floyd Ray stood in the backyard throwing the knife at the ground. Etta came walking through the backyard on her way to the smokehouse carrying a bucket to fill with chicken feed.

Floyd Ray threw the knife towards the ground as Etta walked passed him. Unfortunately, the knife bounced off the ground and thrust into Etta's calf. She instantly dropped her bucket and turned quickly to see what had happened. Blood was running down her leg rapidly. Floyd Ray ran to his grandmother to try and help her get inside. Etta cleaned her wound and applied some healing salve to the cut before wrapping a cloth bandage around the wound. The knife had left a very serious, deep cut to her leg. She probably needed stitches, but she felt she could keep the wound clean and prevent infection from setting in with her own medical supplies.

Floyd Ray felt terrible knowing he had caused his grandmother so much pain. He promised her he would not play with knives anymore. Etta knew it was an accident, although she did scold him for getting the knife in the first place. Floyd Ray learned his lesson about playing with knives that day. He kept his promise—he never played with knives again.

On December 31, 1950, Claude Stokely arrived at Etta's door early in the morning. He was there to bring Etta to deliver his and Bonnie's fourth child. Etta collected her ankle-length coat and medical bag and climbed into the truck with Claude. The cold air whistled through the windows on Claude's truck as he hurried back to his wife with Etta. Claude had to wipe the frost from the windshield every few minutes in order to see the road. He hit several big chuck holes in the dirt road leading to Spicewood Flats, causing Etta to bounce up from her seat, almost hitting her head on the roof of the truck cab. Etta did not say anything to Claude, though—she knew he wanted to get her there as soon as possible in case the baby came quickly.

Claude pulled in the driveway to his home, after what seemed to Etta to be a longer trip than usual, due to the cold and bumpy ride. Etta wrapped her cotton head scarf around her head and pulled her wool coat together tightly as she got out of the truck. The cold wind turned her cheeks and nose a rosy pink as she scurried toward the door of the house.

Etta entered Bonnie's bedroom, where she was lying down. "How are your miseries comin' along now?" Etta asked.

"Well, they're not too bad yet, but I can tell they're gittin' stronger than they wuz," Bonnie answered.

Etta checked Bonnie to find the position of the baby. "Well, everthang seems to be okay. Nothin' to do now, but wait. It'll help you to get up and walk around all you can. Mothers who stay in bed a long time before the real hard miseries start have a harder time, seems like."

Bonnie did as Etta advised, walking through the house from one room to the next until she became too tired to continue. Noon came and went. Etta helped Bonnie prepare the noon meal, then she cleaned up the kitchen after the others had eaten.

Time passed slowly. Nightfall came. Etta started telling about some of her experiences as a midwife to help take Bonnie's mind off her pain. "You know, there was this one couple I was helpin' here awhile back, and the mama didn't seem to want to help push to get the baby to be born. I went in the next room where her husband was, and I told him to go in there and make her real mad.

He said, 'Why, I can't do that to her while she's layin' there 'bout to give birth to our child.' I told him if he wanted that baby to be born, he'd do it! So sure 'nough, he went in there and made her real mad, and do you know that woman had that baby right then and there!" Etta chuckled. Claude and Bonnie loved to sit and listen to Etta's stories, most of which were always amusing.

"The way it's lookin', we might get to bring the 'New Year's Baby' into the world tonight," Etta told Bonnie.

"Law, wouldn't that be somethin' if I wuz the mother of the New Year's baby!" Bonnie said, her eyes sparkling with excitement.

Bonnie started having hard pains around 11:30 P.M. "Okay, it's time to start pushin'," Etta told Bonnie. At 11:59 P.M. a baby girl emerged. "The cord is around her neck. I've got to get it loose!" Etta exclaimed. Etta worked with the baby until she freed the umbilical cord from the baby's neck. She held the baby up by her feet and spanked her on the bottom. The baby started crying instantly. "She'll be okay now," Etta reassured Bonnie with a sigh of relief. "Now, why couldn't you have waited just one more minute?" Etta asked the baby, as she was cleaning her up. "Just one more minute, and I would have got to deliver the New Year's baby," Etta continued. "You have another nine-pounder here," Etta told Bonnie as she weighed the baby. "What 'er you namin' this one?" asked Etta.

"We decided on Wonda Fay Stokely, if it was a girl, so I guess that's what it'll be," answered Bonnie, as she snuggled her little one in her arms.

After staying awhile to make sure Bonnie and the baby were okay, Claude and Etta returned to the truck, and he took her home. It was almost 1:30 A.M. when Etta walked through her front door. She would get only three hours of sleep before time to get up and start another day. She was used to hard work, though. "I wouldn't trade delivering babies for more sleep for no amount of money," Etta thought to herself, as she pulled the $5 Claude had paid her from her coat pocket. Etta put on her warm cotton gown which flowed down to her ankles, then crawled under the pile of colorful homemade quilts she had spent so many days making in previous years. Her head sunk into the fluffy feather pillow as she closed her eyes. At last...her body rested in peaceful slumber.

• • • • • •

On December 30, 1952, June sat on the couch with her son, Tommy, in her arms. Little did she know this would be the last time she would hold her son alive.

Geraldine sat at the kitchen table writing a letter to her cousin, Valerie, while Virginia Ann sat at the table beside her with her coloring book and crayons. John was home on this day doing some work in the basement.

After Tommy fell asleep in her arms, June arose from her seat and laid her son down on the couch. She went into the kitchen and began mopping the floor.

Virginia Ann looked in at Tommy then turned to her mother and said in a slightly frantic tone, "Mama, there's something wrong with Tommy!"

June told Geraldine, "Go to the basement and get your father!" as she ran hurriedly into the living room. When June reached Tommy, it was already too late; her son was dead. He had died from the heart condition he'd had since his birth.

Word spread quickly to the area neighbors and family members about the tragedy of the two-year-old. Mrs. Hash, one of the neighbors, came over and bathed Tommy; he was slightly dirty from playing earlier that day. Soon people started gathering at the Gilliland house to offer their sympathy and support. The kitchen table held food prepared by friends and neighbors. Rev. S. D. Rhoades came as soon as he heard. He walked over to Virginia Ann, knelt down on one knee, and told her, "God is gathering his bouquet, and he needed a little bud."

After the funeral services, Tommy was buried at Jarnigan Cemetery in Morristown. Etta was deeply saddened by the loss of her grandson, but she was never one to question God's will.

It was a cold March day when Datis Cagle drove up to Etta's house to bring her to deliver his and Nancy's first child. They lived in Big Creek, not far from where Harrison and Etta use to live up in the Fifteenth. Etta collected her medical bag and some clothes, for she knew she might be there a few days, then she put on her heavy winter coat before leaving with Datis.

Etta checked Nancy when she got there. "It'll be some time yet. You've not dilated enough to go any time soon," Etta told Nancy.

"You'll stay 'til I'm ready, won't you?" Nancy asked anxiously. "With this bein' my first'n, I want to make sure you're here when I need you," a frightened Nancy continued.

"I'll be right here. You don't have to worry 'bout a thang. Just get up and walk around all you can. It'll make the delivery easier," Etta reassured her.

Three days later, on March 11, 1952, Nancy started having hard "miseries." Nancy was terrified. Nancy's sister, Delia Ball, and Datis were in the room with her and Etta. Datis helped hold Nancy's knees while Delia held her hands. Etta started praying as she prepared for the delivery. After several hours of torturous pain, Nancy gave birth to a 10-pound baby girl. They named her Alberta Cagle. Datis paid Etta $15, then took her home.

A little over one month later, Ben Mooneyham, also from Big Creek, pulled into Etta's driveway. His wife, Jennie Mae was in labor. It seemed to Etta every time the moon turned full she could expect someone to knock on her door in need of a midwife. Once more Etta was off to help bring another baby into the world. At least the weather was warmer now.

Ben and Etta arrived at his home early in the morning. Etta stayed all day with no signs of hard labor from Jennie Mae. Nightfall came. Still Jennie's pains got no stronger. Ben's mother and father were staying with them to help out. They could see Etta was worn out, so they all decided to go to bed early. The next morning on April 21, 1952, Jennie Mae gave birth to a 9-pound baby boy. He was named Walter Don Mooneyham. Ben took Etta home after she concluded mother and baby were both fine. She was paid $10 for her services.

Marie Smith was the daughter of Arthur E. Smith and Leone Smith, Floyd's sister. Marie married Jack Clark, the son of Rev. and Mrs. Homer Clark, who resided in Virginia. Jack and Marie were building a house on the other side of the road across from Floyd and Belle's house in Smithville. Arthur E. and Leone's house stood beside Jack and Marie's, about an acre away. Arthur E. and Jack worked in Akin, South Carolina together. The two families lived there, but often came to Del Rio to visit with relatives. On this particular visit, Leone was very excited because she had won a television set in a drawing at a grocery store in Akin. No one Leone knew in Del Rio owned a television set. They brought the TV home with them to Smithville, anxious to get the antenna hooked to it so they could relax and enjoy the programs.

Belle sat in a chair on her screened-in back porch shelling peas as she watched Jack Clark climb the hillside behind her house. He was going to place the antenna at the top of the hill so he could get the best possible reception for his mother-in-law. Jack threw the television wire across some power lines before he crossed the creek on his way back to Leone and Arthur E.'s house. After wading through the creek, Jack bent down and picked up the antenna wire.

Linda, who would be five the next month, was playing in her front yard when she noticed Jack's body beginning to smoke. Jack was being electrocuted before young Linda's eyes! Linda ran around the house to her mother on the back porch. "Mama, Jack Clark's a-smokin'!" shouted Linda excitedly. Belle did not give any special attention to her daughter's remark because she thought Linda was referring to Jack smoking a cigarette. Soon Belle began to hear a loud commotion across the road. She removed the pan of peas from her lap and walked to the front of the house to see what was going on. There Belle saw Arthur E. with a wooden chair in his hand trying desperately to knock the live wires out of Jack's hand. Just then Floyd and his brother, Arthur B., pulled in Floyd's driveway as they returned home from their job at Enka. Just as Floyd was getting out of the car, Arthur E. opened the back door and laid Jack in the back seat. Arthur E. jumped in the front seat next to Arthur B. "We gotta get Jack to the hospital! He's been electrocuted!" Arthur E. shouted. Arthur B. scowled his tires as he took off down the road. Unfortunately, they were too late—Jack died just as Arthur B. was turning onto Highway 107, about two miles away from Smithville.

Marie was pulling into her driveway as Arthur B. and Arthur E. started down the road with Jack. She had been to the funeral of one of her friends. Leone consoled her daughter as she told her the devastating news about her husband. Marie held her and Jack's 17-month-old baby boy, Marty, tightly in her arms as the shocking news began to sink in. Tears filled her eyes as she prayed for her husband.

When Belle learned about the horrible tragedy which had taken place across the road from her house, she went immediately up to her mother's to tell her about the horrible incident. Etta cried tears of sorrow upon hearing the awful news about Jack. Her heart went out to Marie and her son.

Jack Clark died on September 16, 1953, at the age of 25. Funeral services were held at The First Church of God, just below Smithville. Rev. James I. Turner performed the ceremony. Jack's body was laid to rest in the Clark Cemetery on Midway road.

Etta continued going on several baby cases each month. People who used her services in the past kept calling on her about every two years. They also came to her when they got sick to get a shot, or to get some medicine. Etta began giving shots with a hypodermic needle when she realized the need for a "country doctor" in the area. A lot of people in the surrounding communities were still very poor and could not afford to pay the doctors in Newport.

Etta kept penicillin, teramycin, erythromycin, and tetracycline antibiotics. She gave big, red kidney pills to people with kidney problems, and kept sinus pills on hand for people with sinusitis. Etta made her own cough remedy with honey and lemon juice, and, of course, there was nothing like a good cleaning out using good ole Castoria, a very harsh, but effective laxative.

Etta bought her medical supplies from a pharmacy in Newport at a special discount, because the pharmacist knew she was a country doctor for people in Cocke County, Tennessee, and Madison County, North Carolina.

The people who used her services thought she was the best doctor around, and they kept coming back. Soon Etta's home was a busy place with patients coming and going to get this remedy, or that remedy for "whatever ailed them."

Harrison was very understanding through all the comings and goings of the people invading his home. He never complained...much. He realized this was Etta's "calling," so he did not try to stand in her way. The people needed her, and he knew it. He even pitched in and helped Etta fill out the birth certificates and the necessary paper work on her patients. Most men would not have tolerated having their home turned into a busy medical office, but Harrison always showed great patience with Etta and accepted it all as their way of life.

On May 19, 1954, Etta's 57th birthday, Emily came to stay with her mother to give birth to her fourth child. Oh, how excited Etta was, to think her grandchild might be born on her birthday, and she would get to deliver it, too! Unfortunately, Etta's birthday passed without Emily giving birth.

Valerie and Sandra made a bed on the couch in the living room. Emily slept in the back bedroom just off from the kitchen. Etta laid down in her bed which occupied one side of the living room. Soon everyone was asleep.

In the early morning hours, Emily quietly awakened her mother. "It's time, Mama," Emily whispered as she gently shook her mother. Etta sprang from her bed and followed Emily into the back bedroom. Valerie and Sandra slept on. Emily gave birth to a baby boy on the morning of May 20, 1954. Emily wanted to name her son after the preacher at Round Mountain Baptist church, Darrell Seals, but she would wait on Dick to arrive before deciding on anything definite.

The morning brought bright sunshine beaming into the living room where Valerie and Sandra slept. They rubbed their sleepy eyes and stretched their arms over their head as they got out of bed. Sandra walked into the back bedroom where her mother and grandmother were. Much to Sandra's surprise, her mother had another baby in her arms! This did not go over too well with Sandra—she was supposed to be the baby! She ran and jumped on the bed, crawling over top of her newborn brother into her mother's arms. Sandra started crying as she pleaded with her mother, "Can't you take it back? Can't you please take it back?!"

Etta shook in laughter as she quickly pulled her granddaughter off the baby and Emily.

Valerie liked her new brother; she just wondered where in the world he had come from; he was not there when she went to sleep the night before. Dick arrived at Etta's shortly after the two sisters met their little brother. Dick was thrilled to learn he had a son. Emily told him she wanted to name him Darrell.

"Well, we'll call him Darrell if you will also add Charles, after my boss," Dick answered. They also wanted to name him after his father, so the name; Charles Richard Darrell Jones was agreed upon by the two proud parents.

On June 23, 1954, Belle went into labor with her fourth child. Floyd drove up to Etta's to get her to come perform the delivery. It was early in the day, around 9:00 A.M. when Etta arrived to care for Belle at her home in Smithville.

Floyd stayed in the room with Belle this time, holding her hands whenever the pains became strong. He had not been present for the birth of any of their previous children.

Belle's water broke around 2:00 P.M., but the baby did not come until several hours later. "This is gonna be a dry birth, Belle. Your 'miseries' will be worse with this one than they were with the others, so you'll have to muster

Etta "Granny" Nichols—Last of the Old-Timey Midwives

up all the strength you got to push the baby out," Etta prepared her daughter.

"I feel like I need to go to the bathroom," Belle said. Floyd and Etta helped Belle out of bed and to the bathroom. Belle barely made it back to the bed before the baby came. It was a girl.

Witnessing the pain of childbirth proved too much for Floyd. He walked over to the doorway and started to cry. After he composed himself, Floyd came back in to get another look at his new daughter. She weighed 10-pounds, had almost no hair, except for one little curl on top, and had her daddy's blue eyes. Floyd and Belle named their new addition Venida Ellen Smith. Etta stayed with Belle that night before she went home. She came back each day for the next several days until Belle was able to do for herself and her family.

Floyd Ray stayed with Etta quite frequently when he was a baby. Etta felt very close to him, and he to her, since she practically raised him during the first few years of his life. She wanted Belle to leave Floyd Ray with her when he was a baby, maybe because she felt her daughter was too inexperienced to care for a baby properly, and she loved having a baby in her home to care for.

Because of the bond Floyd Ray shared with his grandparents, he visited them very often. One day while Floyd Ray was visiting, Harrison put the mule in a harness and was leading it from the barn to the field below the house to do some plowing. Floyd Ray walked out on the back porch when he saw his grandfather coming from the barn with the mule. The mule got to an area between the house and the chicken coop and realized where Harrison was taking him. The mule decided it was not in the mood to do any plowing this day. It bowed up and would not move an inch. Harrison took the leather straps on the harness and whipped the mule as hard as he could. Oh, he was furious with that mule! The mule did not budge. Harrison walked over and picked up a big stick and hit the mule right between the eyes with a hard blow. The mule jumped back and let out a loud bray...then it went! The mule minded Harrison from then on.

Floyd Ray ran inside to tell his grandmother of what he had witnessed. "I thought he was going to kill it, as hard as he hit it. I ain't never seen Poy (the name Floyd Ray called his grandfather) that mad before," Floyd Ray exclaimed.

"Well, mules get contrary from time to time. You have to let 'em know who's boss. The mule will be okay," Etta chuckled.

Etta's next grandchild, unfortunately, was stillborn when June gave birth to her fourth baby on April 23, 1955, at Morristown-Hamblen Hospital. Dr. Roach performed the delivery. It saddened the doctor to inform the excited parents of the baby's fate. They named their little girl Mary Gilliland. John and June would try again. John hoped for another son, especially since he had lost Tommy.

Thirteen months later June went to Morristown-Hamblen Hospital once more. She was in labor with her fifth child. Dr. Zimmerman would perform the delivery. June had not been in the delivery room long when a nurse came out to inform John, "You're the father of a healthy baby girl." Though John was somewhat disappointed, he would love his daughter no less than if she had been a boy. John and June named their little girl Johnnie Sue Gilliland. She looked like her oldest sister, Geraldine, with dark curly hair, and beautiful brown eyes. She only missed her sister's birthday by 12 days. Geraldine was born on May 12th; Johnnie Sue was born on May 24, 1956.

One year passed before Etta had another grandchild to enter the world. On May 11, 1957, Belle went into labor with her fifth child. Floyd had not come home from work yet, so Marie Smith Clark drove Belle to Valentine-Shults Hospital in Newport. Mary Bell Smith, Floyd's sister-in-law, rode with Marie and Belle, also. It was almost 9 P.M. when the women reached the hospital. Belle was placed in a room just across the hall from the nursery. She shared the room with Mrs. Edith Barrett, wife of Jack Barrett. Earlier that day, Edith had given birth to a son, whom they named Donald.

Belle had experienced false labor two weeks earlier. She went to her mother thinking she was in labor. Etta gave Belle some castor oil to help bring on the "miseries." This made Belle's pains worse, but no baby came. Dr. Shults had been monitoring Belle's pregnancy this time because he was afraid she would not be able to carry the baby through full-term.

When Floyd came home he took the other children to Etta's then he left to go be with his wife. The next day, on May 12, 1957, also Mother's Day, Belle was wheeled into the delivery room just before noon. When she came out she held a new baby girl. Floyd and Belle named their daughter, Sharon Kay Smith. She weighed 10-pounds, had a full head of brown, curly hair, and her daddy's blue eyes.

Sharon appeared much larger than the other 6- and 7-pound babies in the nursery. People standing at the nursery window looked at all the babies, then turned and looked into Belle's room. Belle felt they must be fascinated with the woman who gave birth to this large baby, but a lot of women from the mountains gave birth to large babies. It must have been the good, wholesome food the country people ate, coming from their own gardens.

Belle told Floyd, "This was the easiest labor of any of my previous deliveries. Mrs. Zimmery Ball put me to sleep before the pains became too strong. When I woke up the baby had come."

Floyd stood in the doorway with a look of disappointment on his face. Belle felt that he had secretly been hoping for another son. This would be the last child Floyd and Belle would have because Dr. Shults felt Belle should not have any more children, due to health reasons.

It was a warm spring day in 1957 when Loiree and her son, Michael walked down to her sister's, Iva Smith Freeman, who lived across the road from their mother, Mary Smith, in Smithville. Loiree sent seven-year-old Michael outside to play while she helped Iva varnish a dresser inside the house. Iva and her husband, Boyd, were building a new house on some property behind Mary's house.

Novie was walking down the road going back to her house located at the beginning of Midway Road when she passed Iva's house and saw Michael playing in the yard. Novie decided she would go inside and visit with Loriee and Iva before going on home. She went in the bedroom where the two women were working and sat down on a box of quilts Iva had sitting on the floor. Novie had not been there long when Michael came running through the door with a nosebleed. When Novie saw her grandson with blood all over his face, she stood up in a panic and shouted, "Lordy mercy!" as she threw her hands up in the air. When Novie brought her arms down, she lost her balance and fell backwards over the box of quilts she had been sitting on. Novie could not get up—she had broken her hip!

The doctor did not give any hope to Etta that her mother's hip would mend; after all, Novie was eighty years old. Novie would spend the rest of her days confined to her bed. But Novie refused to move in with any of her children—she was not leaving her home!

Loiree drove up to Etta's each morning to give her a ride to Novie's house so she could tend to her mother. In the evening Loiree went back to pick Etta up and take her back home.

Novie's children worried about her being alone for any long period of time, so it was decided Chan Smith would be hired to build a small house for Novie beside Lurlie and Iowa up the road in London. Lurlie could check on his mother from time to time during the hours Etta was not there.

J. L. paid for the construction of his mother's new house. Chan had the house finished just as fall arrived. Lurlie also helped Chan with the construction of his mother's house. It had one large front room with the kitchen on the right-hand side as one entered the front door, On the left side of the room, a door provided the

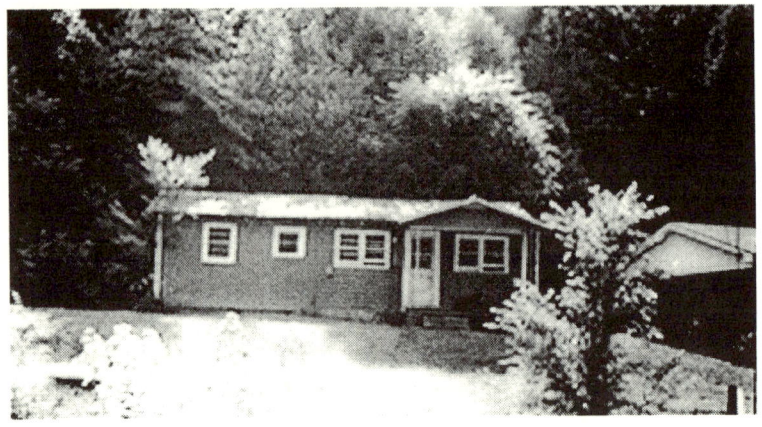

Novie Grigsby's House

entrance to a large bedroom. Etta later had a small bathroom added in one corner of the bedroom. The bedroom had a door which led outside. There was also a door at the back of the house next to the kitchen.

Novie was moved into her new house by her children. Her bed was placed in the front room under the windows at the front of the house. Etta placed a bed for herself in the bedroom. She would be staying with her mother during the nights now and going back home during the day.

Etta's first grandchild, Valerie, had married James David "Bunton" Thornton during the first part of 1957. At age 16, Valerie was due to have her first child in mid-December. Valerie went to stay with her mother, Emily, a couple of weeks before the baby was due in order to get to the clinic quicker than she could from her house in Chestnut Hill.

On December 16, 1957, Valerie was taken to Dr. Nease's clinic in Newport to give birth. Emily went into the delivery room with her daughter. When Emily came out, she was the proud grandmother of a baby girl. She weighed 9-pounds and 3-ounces and had flame-red hair all over her head, and pretty blue eyes.

When Bunton saw his little girl for the first time, he walked over to Valerie in her hospital bed and said, "You had us the purttiest little redheaded girl." Valerie looked up and smiled pleasingly at Bunton.

The two proud parents named their firstborn Vicki Jean Thornton. Etta was now a great-grandmother at the age of 60.

Almost two months had passed since Valerie gave birth to Vicki. She had not been able to take her daughter to meet her great-grandmother Nichols due to the cold, harsh winter weather. Now that the weather was more favorable, Valerie, Emily, and Vicki finally were able to go visit Etta. Oh, Etta "pitched a fit" over her first great-grandchild. She could not get over how red her hair was. Etta held Vicki for a long time before putting her back in Valerie's arms.

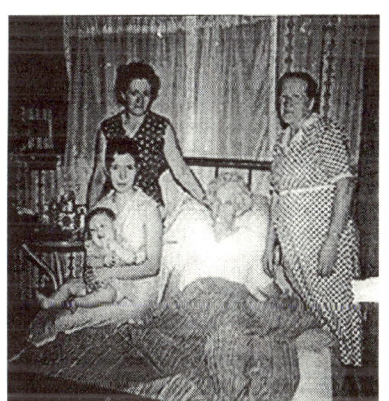

Left standing: Emily Jones. Right standing: Etta Nichols. Sitting: Valerie holds her daughter, Vicki. Novie lies in bed

Before Emily, Valerie, and Vicki left to go back to their homes, they went to visit Novie. While there, they had a picture made of the five generations standing together around Novie's bed. This was a picture Vicki could have to cherish when she grew up.

Etta continued delivering babies between the births of her grandchildren. On January 27, 1958, Ben Mooneyham came to Etta's house to take her to his wife, Jennie Mae, who was in labor with their third child. Etta had delivered their previous two children also. Her last visit to the Mooneyham home was rewarded by delivering a healthy 9 1/2-pound baby boy on March 1, 1954. Ben and Jennie Mae named him Dan Reed Mooneyham. Their first child was Walter Don Mooneyham, born on April 21, 1952.

It was late in the evening when Etta arrived to deliver a third child for the Mooneyhams. In the early morning hours, on January 28, Jennie Mae gave birth to another healthy baby boy. He weighed 10 1/4-pounds. Etta had mentioned her grandsons name previously to the Mooneyhams. They liked it so much they named their son after him: Floyd Ray Mooneyham. Grandpa and Grandma Mooneyham were there to help with the other children and the chores, so when daybreak came Ben took Etta back to her house. Ben had just reached Etta's house when the snow began to pour down. Etta snuggled up next to the coal fire Harrison had built in the fireplace and took a short nap before starting her daily chores.

In February 1959, Emily went to her mother's to stay during the last two months of her pregnancy. Valerie stayed with her dad to help with the children and other household chores. Emily was not physically able to do the housework and take care of her other children, being seven months pregnant. Two months after Emily went to

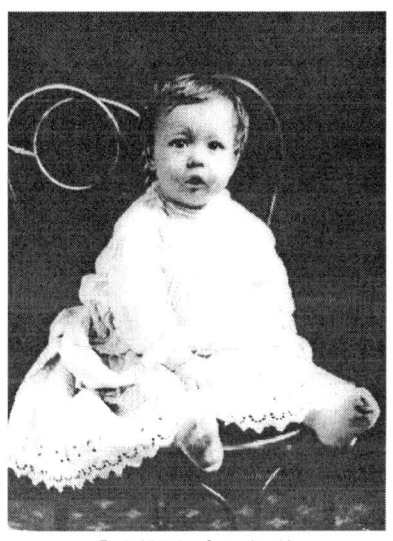

Emily Nichols—9 months old

her mother's, she gave birth to a baby girl on April 14, 1959.

Etta had a baby picture of Emily on the wall over the bed where Emily was sleeping.

When Dick, Valerie, and the other children came to meet the new family member, Valerie commented to her mother that the baby looked just like she did in the picture on the wall. Dick and Emily's last child was named, Debra Eilene Jones. This baby would be Etta's last grandchild.

More Photos

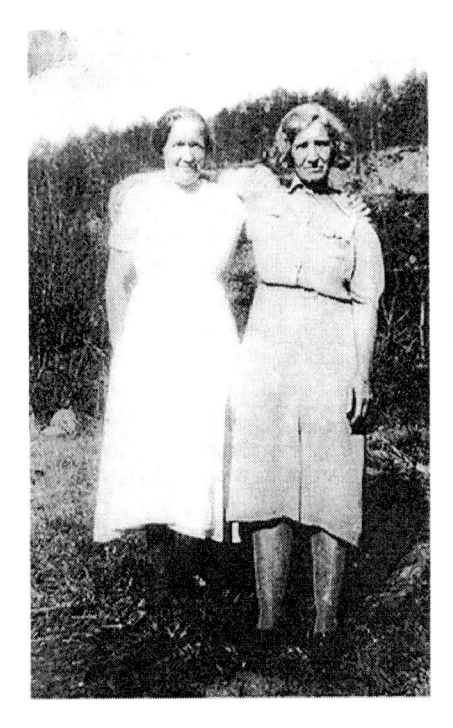

Etta Grigsby Nichols in her mid-twenties, and mother, Nova Grigsby—Early 1920s.

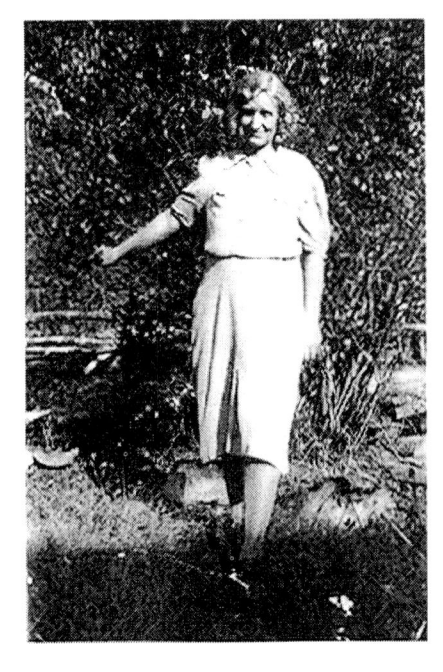

Nova Grigsby—Early 1920s.

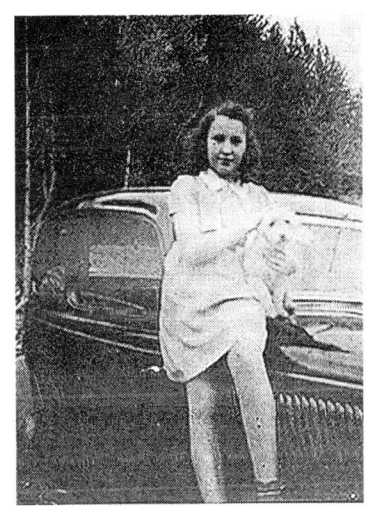

Belle Nichols, 11 years old, and her dog, Bootie.

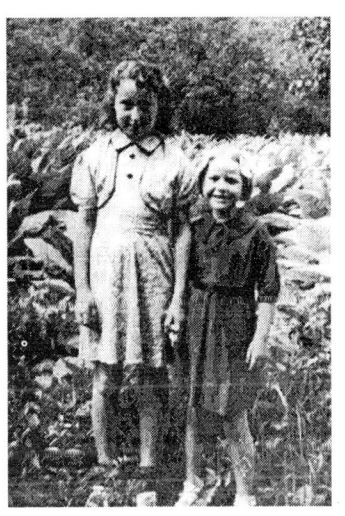

Belle Nichols, 8 years old, and friend.

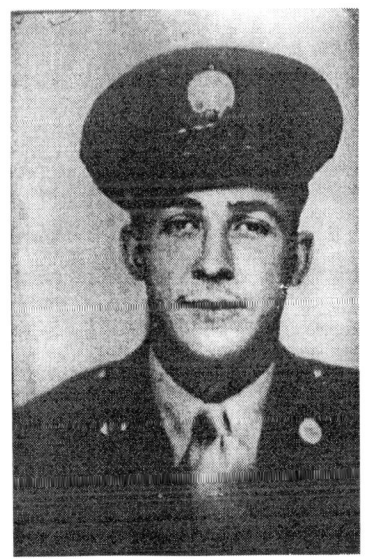

John Thomas Gilliland—Age 21

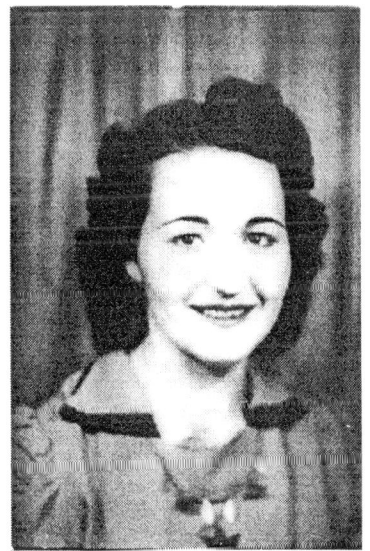

June Nichols—Age 19

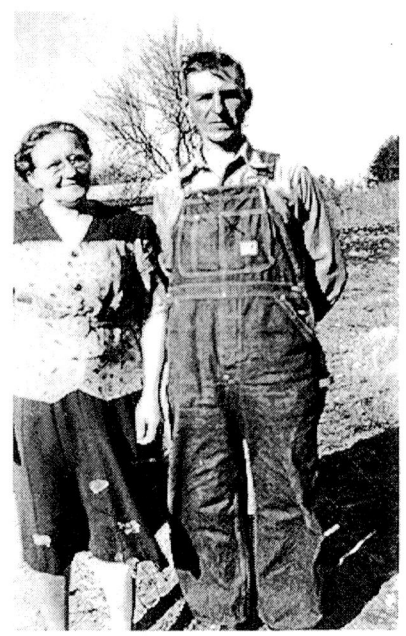

Harrison and Etta Nichols—Spring 1946.

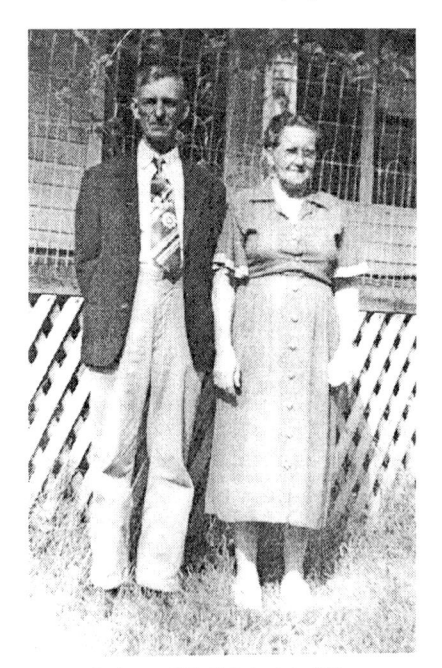

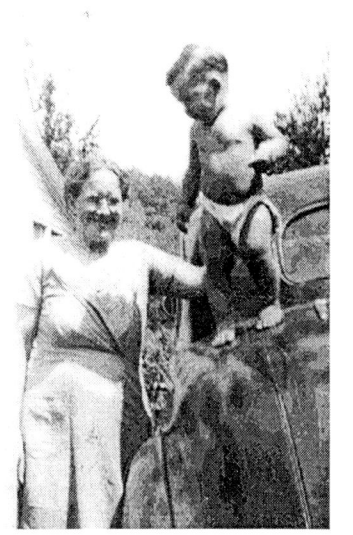

Etta Nichols and Floyd Ray—Age 1

Harrison and Etta Nichols—Late 1950s.

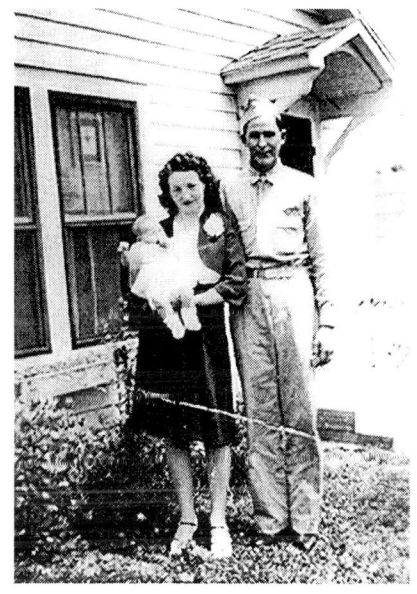

John & June Gilliland and daughter,
Geraldine—Fall of 1942

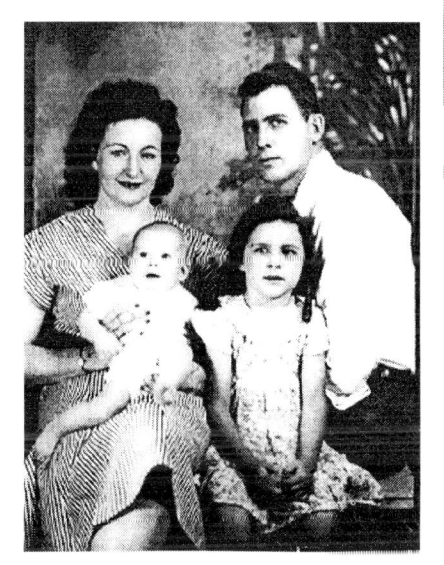

John Thomas Gilliland in uniform

John, June, Geraldine, and Virginia Ann
Gilliland—1947

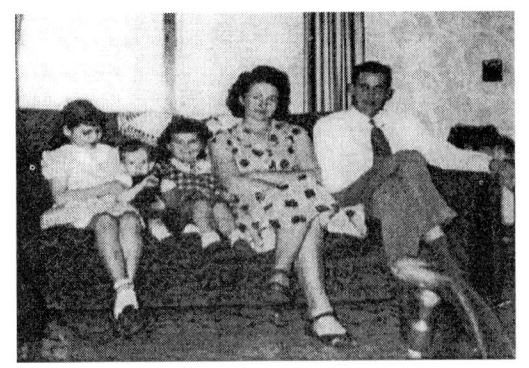

From right: John, June, Virginia Ann, Tommy & Geraldine Gilliland—1951

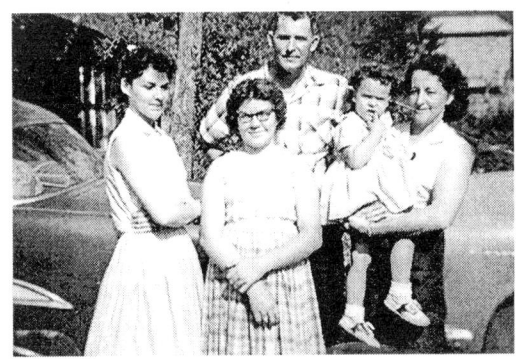

From left: Geraldine, Virginia Ann, John, Johnnie Sue, and June Gilliland

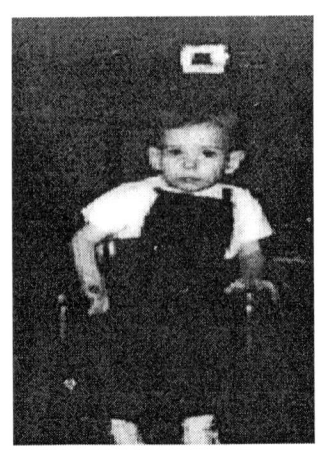

Tommy Gilliland sits in his little rocking chair—1951

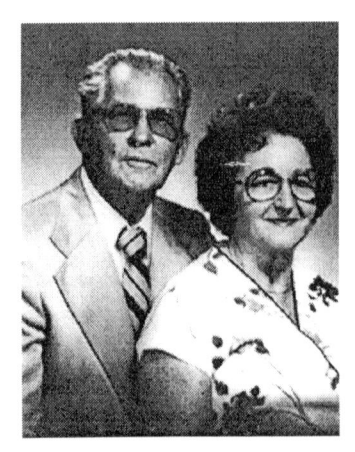

John and June Gilliland's 40th wedding anniversary picture—8-16-1981

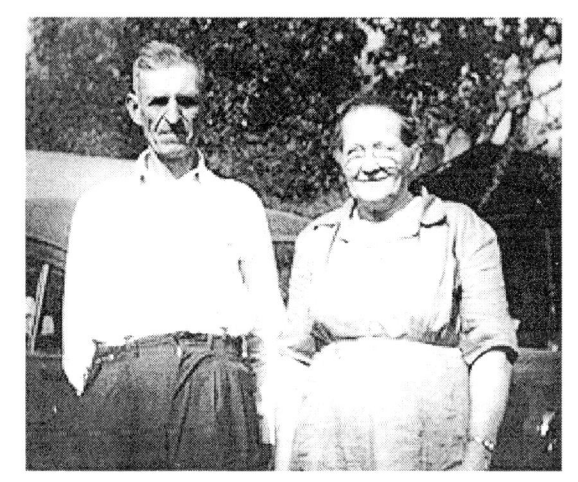

Harrison and Etta Nichols—
May 1959

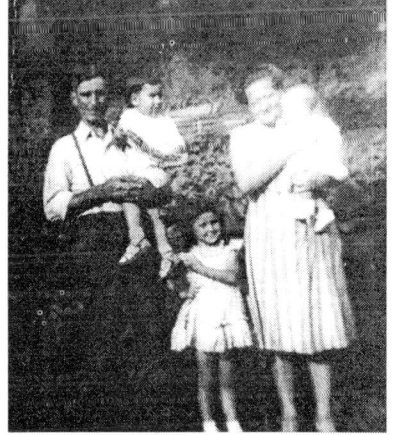

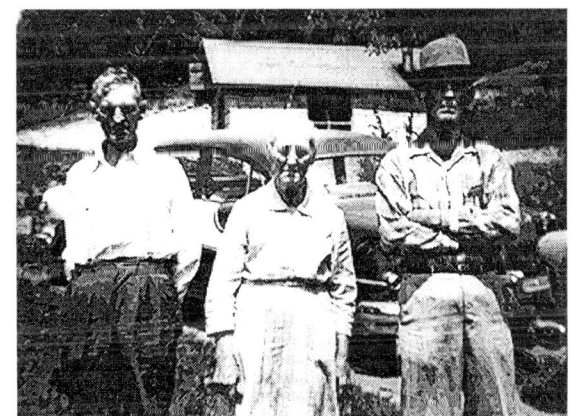

Harrison holds Floyd Ray, Etta holds Virginia Ann.
Standing: Geraldine—1947

From left: Harrison Nichols with Mother, Martha Crowder, and half-brother, Roy Crowder.

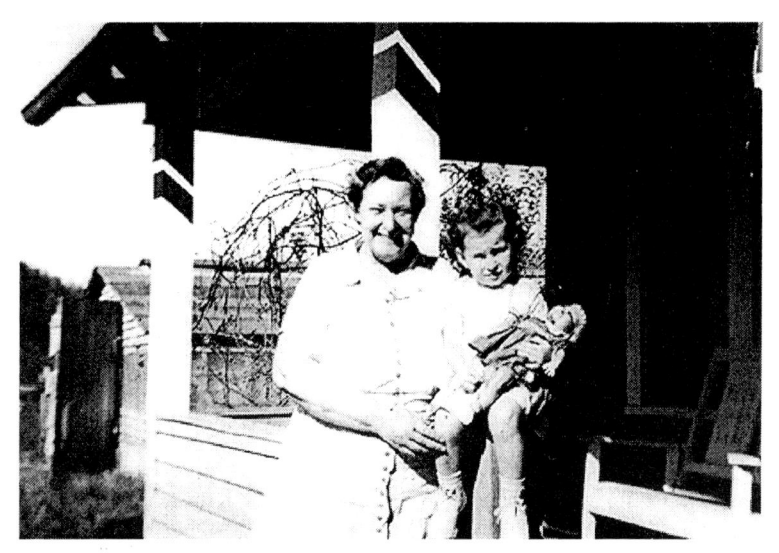

Alverta Taylor, Etta's sister, holds Venida at Floyd and Belle's house in Smithville—1957

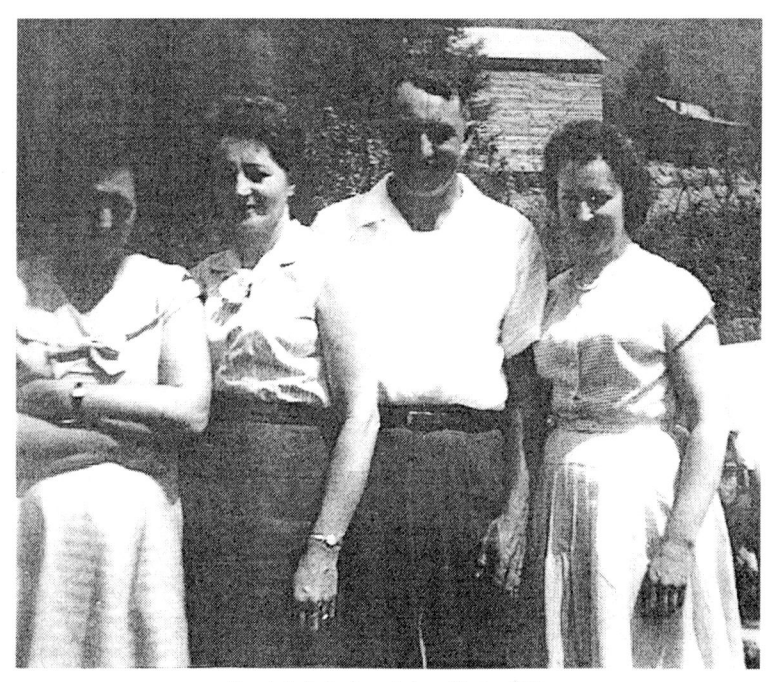

From left: Emily, June, Jack, and Belle—1958

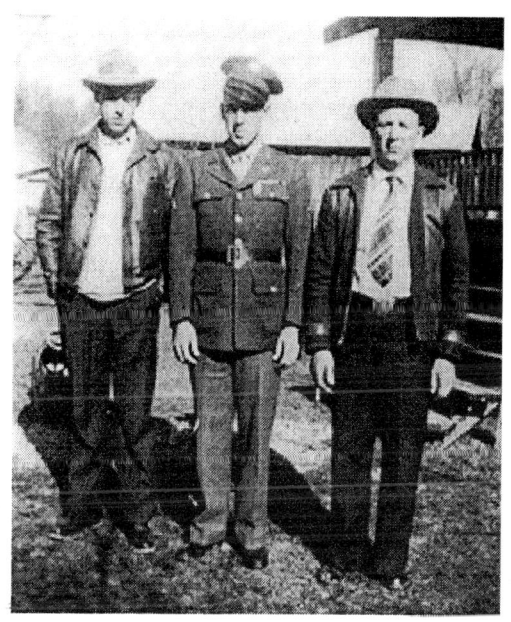

Arthur B. Smith, Floyd J. Smith, and Doyle Smith—1944

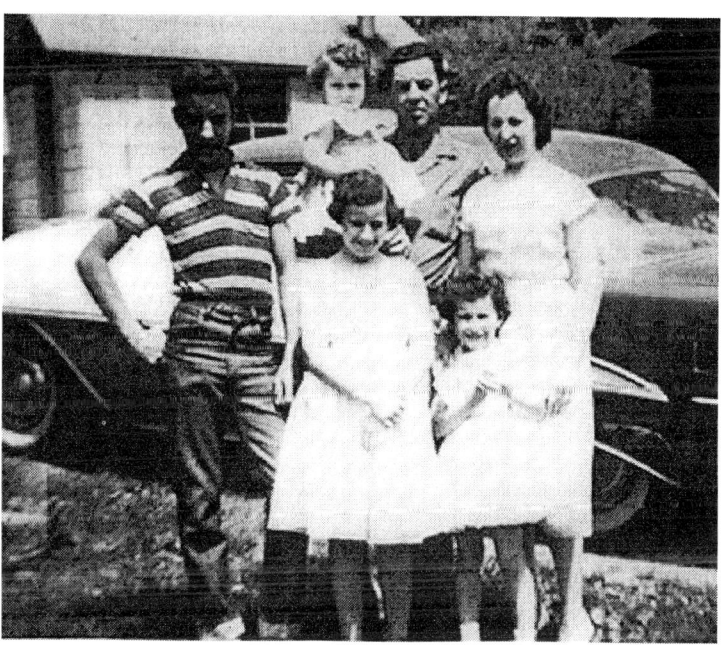

Floyd and Belle Smith's family. From left, top row: Floyd Ray, Floyd J. holds Sharon Kay, Belle. Bottom: Linda and Venida

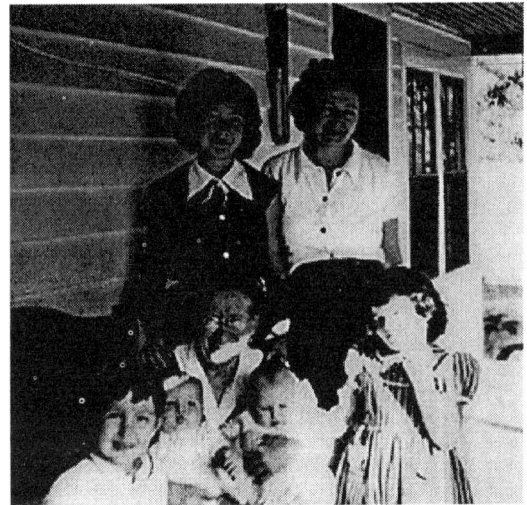

Standing: Emily and Valerie Jones. Sitting, from left: Sandra Jones, Etta holds Darrell and Venida, Linda Smith.

Debbie Jones and Sharon Smith—April 1962

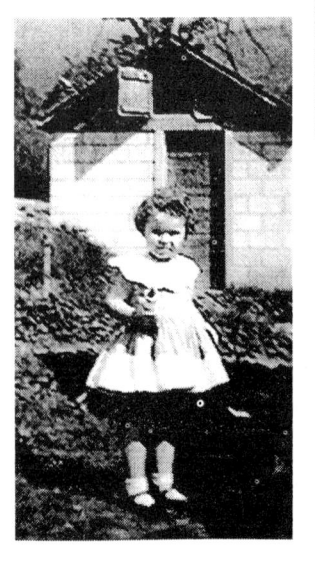

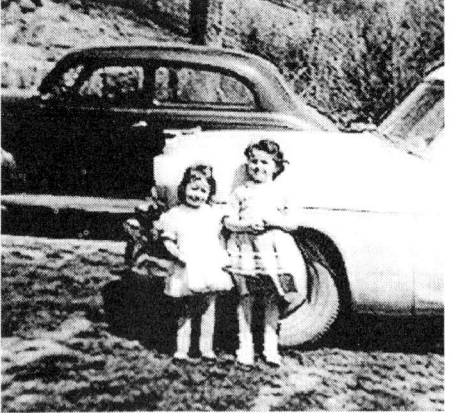

Sharon Smith at Etta's house—Age 2 1/2

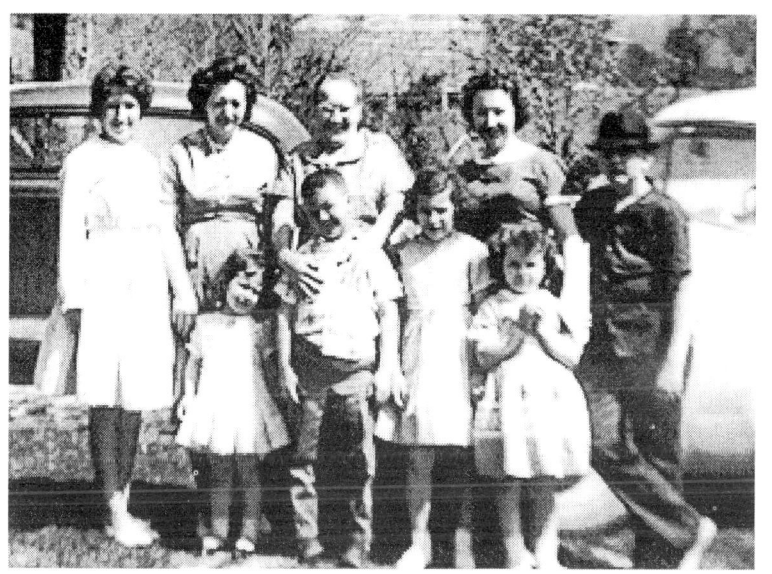

From left—top row: Sandra Jones, Emily Jones, Etta Nichols, Belle Smith, Jimmy Nichols. Bottom row: Debbie Jones, Darrell Jones, Venida Smith, and Sharon Smith—Easter Sunday, April 1962

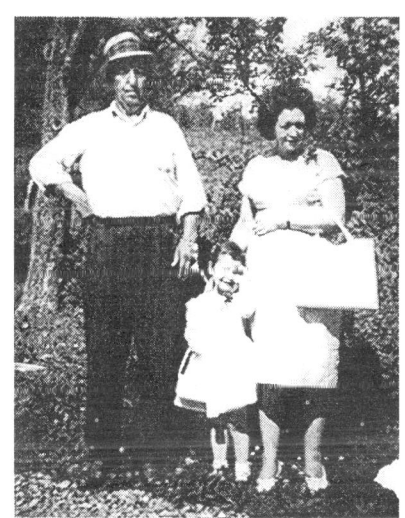

Dick, Emily, and Debbie Jones—May 1962

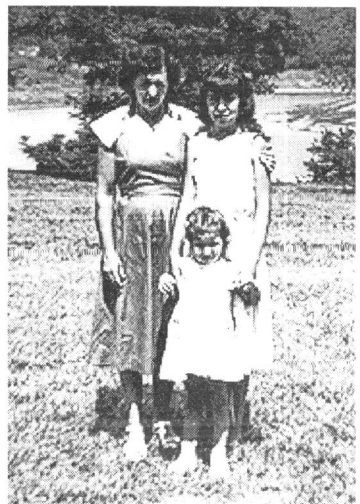

Emily, Valerie, and Sandra Jones—1953

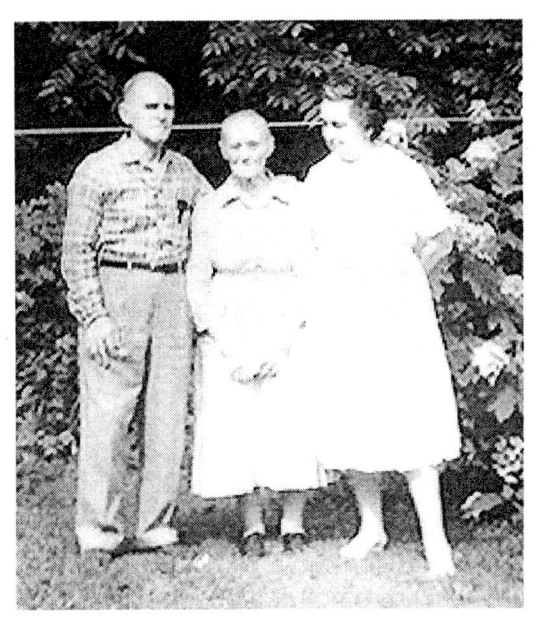

From left: Harrison's only full brother, Claude Nichols, stands with mother, Martha Crowder, and Claude's wife, Ruby—August 1961

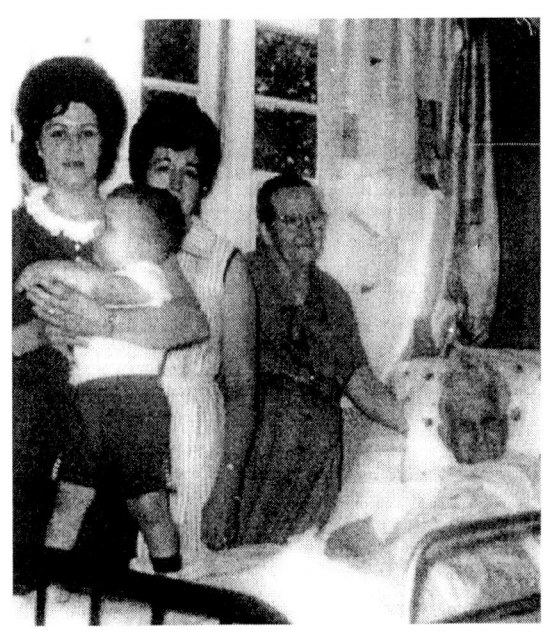

Five generations are shown in this photo of Nova, Etta, June, Geraldine, and her son, John Marco Wall

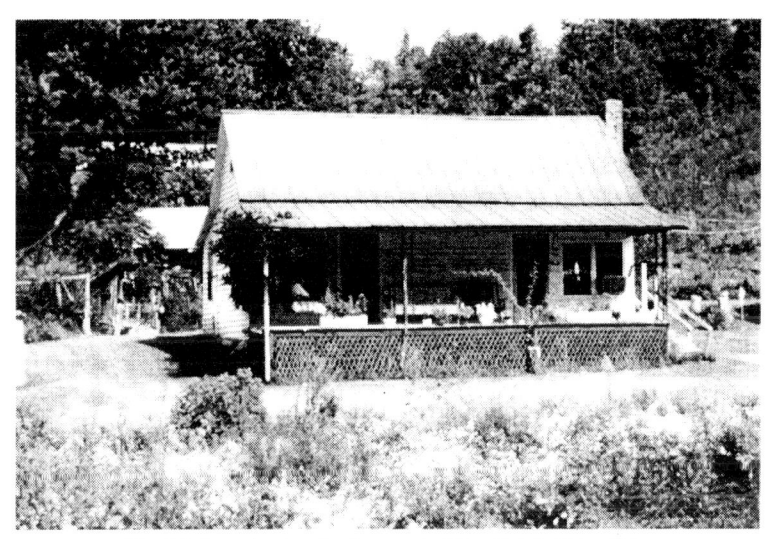

Etta sits in the porch swing at her house, early 1980s. Photo by Michael Sylva

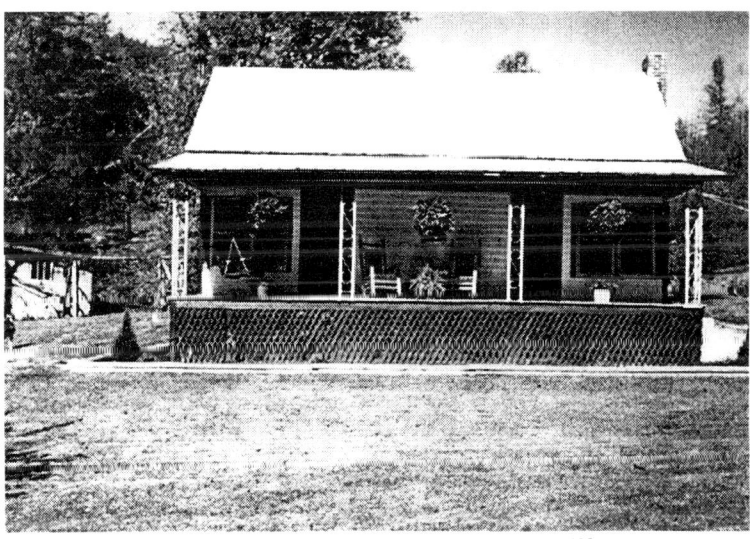

The house formerly owned by Etta Nichols as it appeared in 1996.

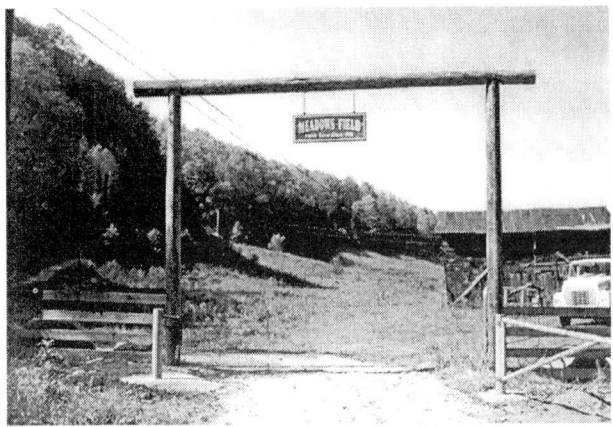

Entrance to Meadows Field as it appeared in 1996. Meadows Field was once owned by John Lewis Grigsby, Etta's father.

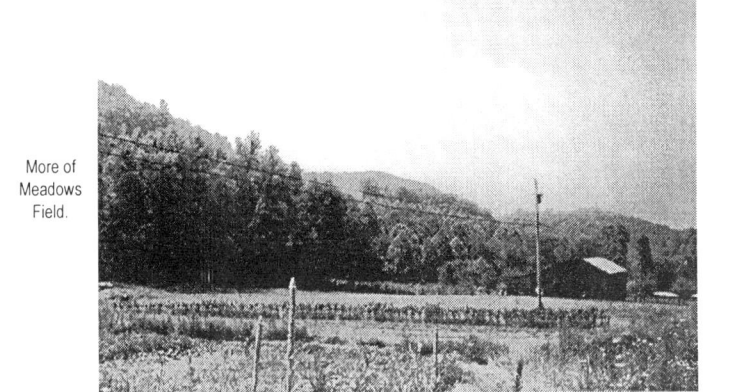

More of Meadows Field.

Some of the beautiful scenery found in Del Rio, along South Hwy. 107. The Round Mountain boasts in majestic splendor as it peaks over the lower mountains.

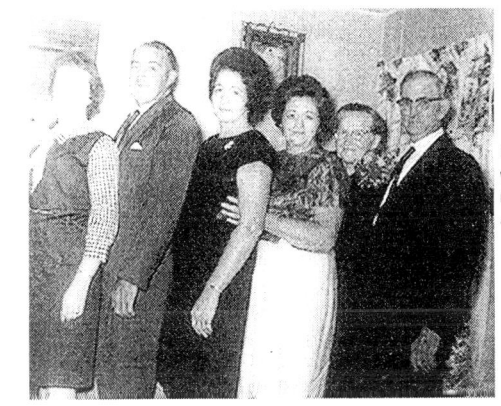

Etta and Harrison celebrate their 50th wedding anniversary at their home. From right: Harrrison, Etta, Emily, June, Jack, and Belle—October 1966.

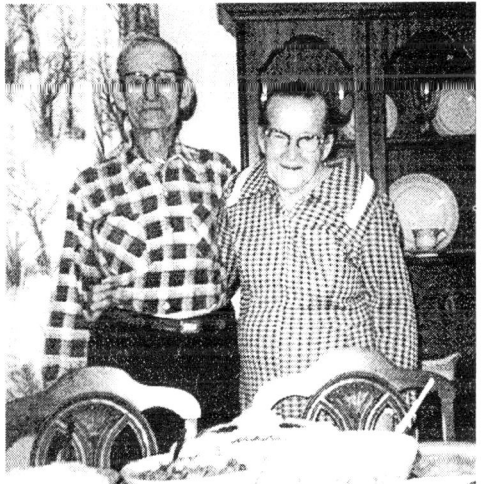

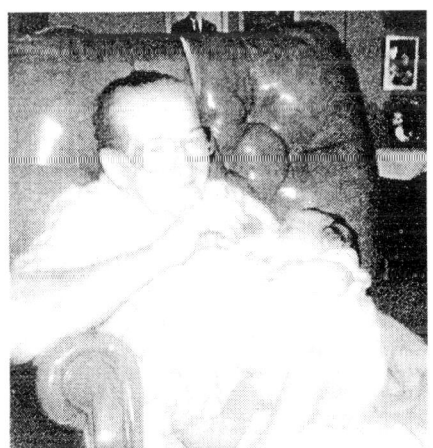

Etta puts her arm around Harrison as they celebrate his birthday, at Belle's house.

Etta holds her great-granddaughter, Amanda, Venida's baby—1984.

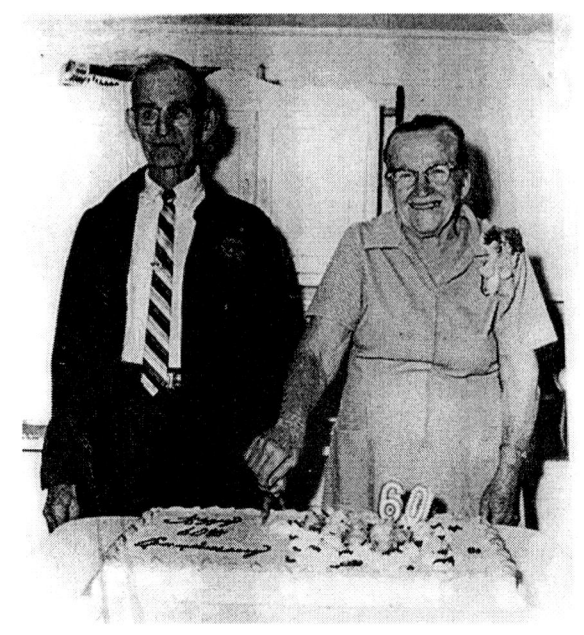

Harrison and Etta celebrate their 60th wedding anniversary. These photos appeared in The Newport Plain Talk with the story of their anniversary.

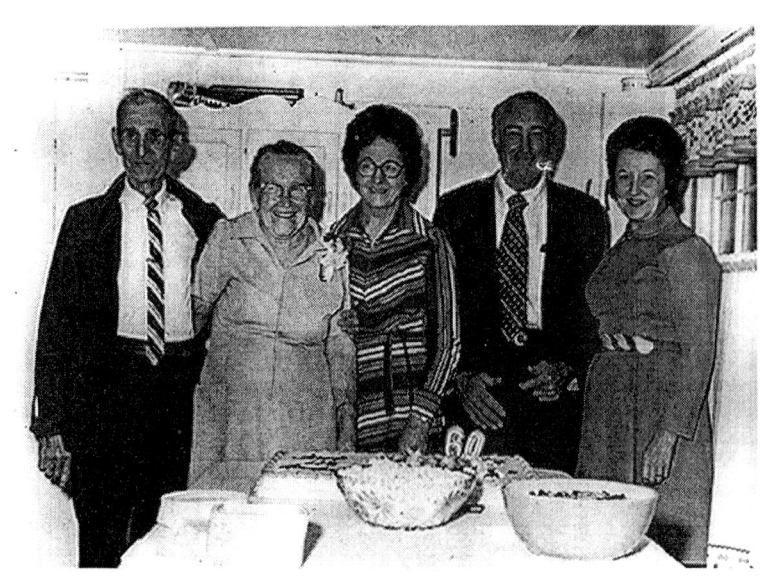

Harrison, Etta, June, Jack, and Belle stand at Etta's table to pose for The Newport Plain Talk Newspaper.

Photos courtesy of: The Newport Plain Talk

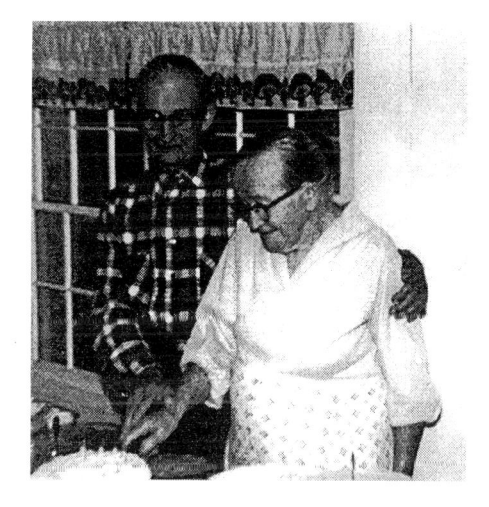

Harrison and Etta celebrate a wedding anniversary.

From left: Etta's brothers, Furman and Lurlie attended the celebration along with Etta's sister, Willie (Bill).

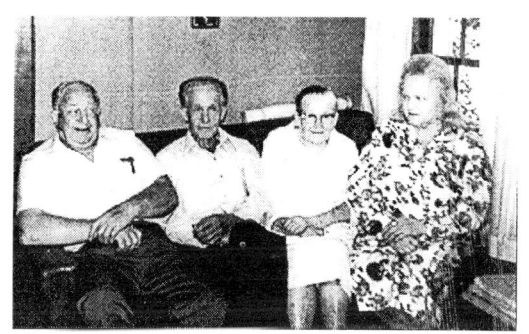

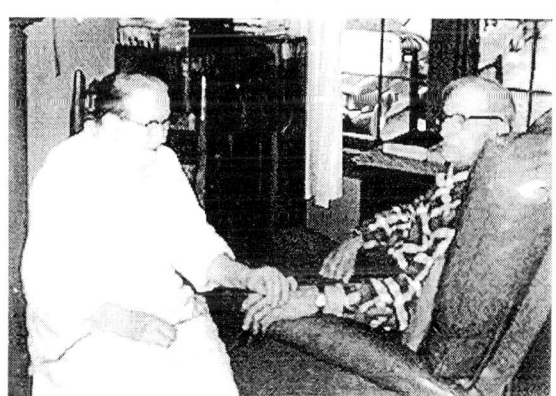

Etta and Harrison show affection for one another after the meal, as they relax in their living room.

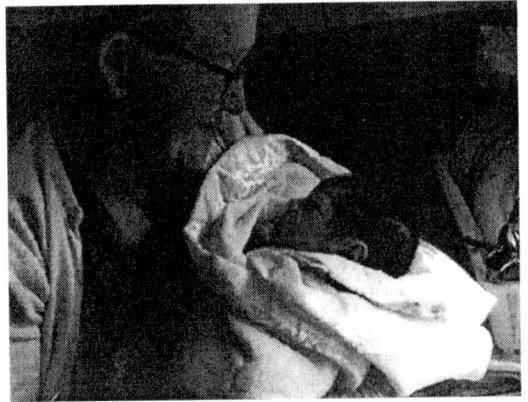

Etta holds one of her deliveries affectionately in her kitchen.

Another delivery Etta holds proudly as she stands barefoot in the grass outside her house.

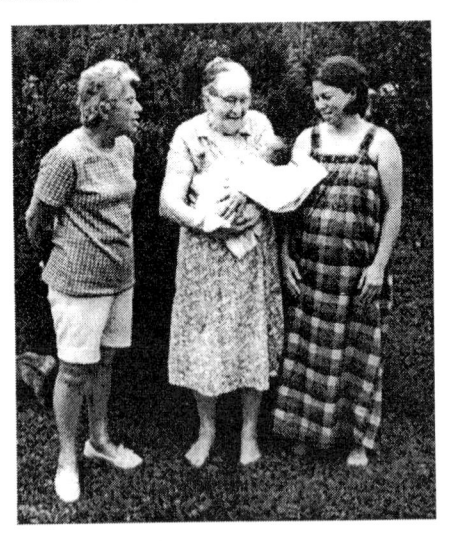

Etta sits in her "baby room" with a new mom and her baby.

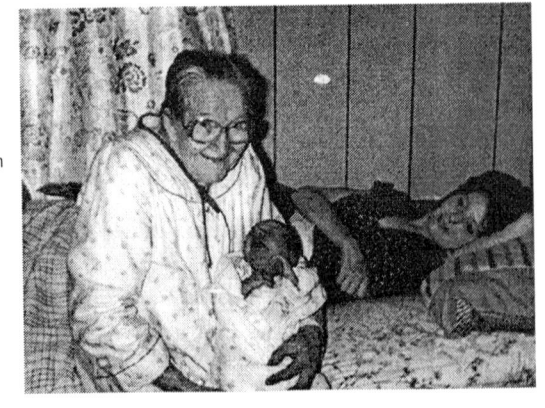

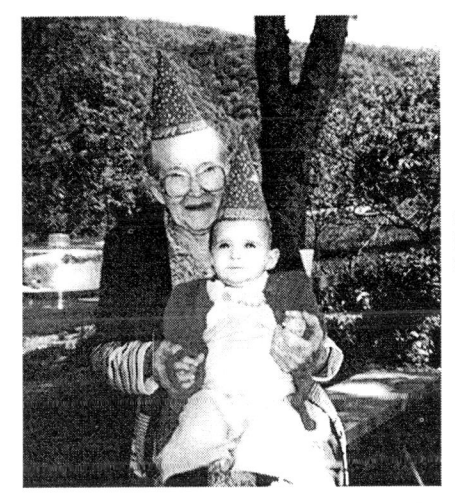

Etta holds Amanda Guillot on her lap as she joins in the celebration of her great-granddaughter's first birthday at Belle's house—July 25, 1985.

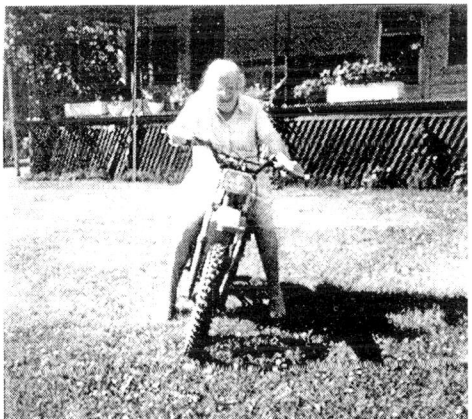

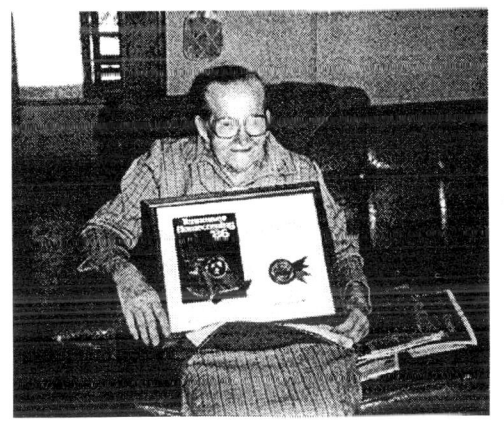

Etta shows that life doesn't have to be over just because you're in your eighties.

Etta holds her 1986 homecoming award as she sits in her living room.

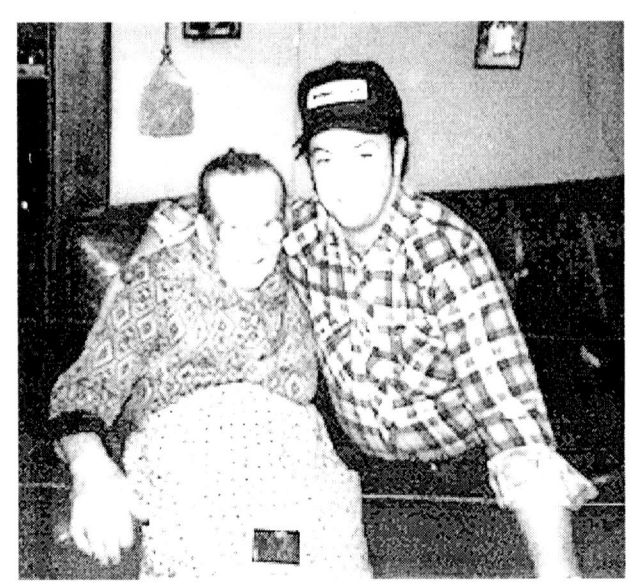

Darrell Jones gets an affectionate hug from his grandmother as they pose on her couch.

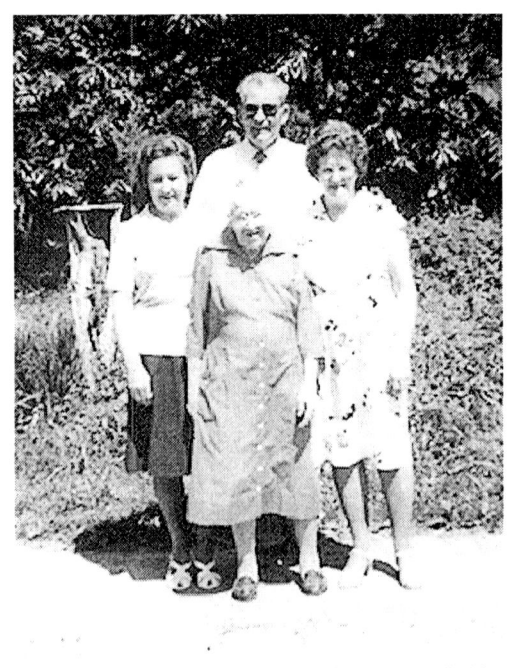

John and June Gilliland pose with Etta. Belle Smith stands on the left.

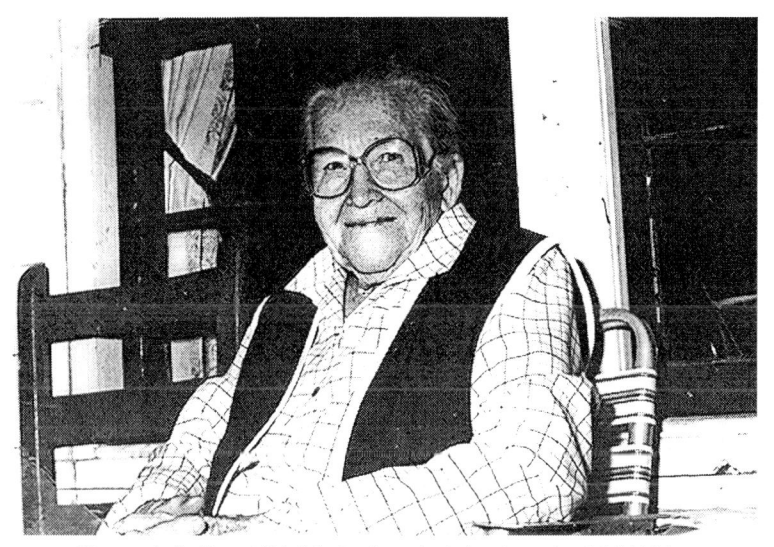

Etta poses for the Newport Plain Talk when they arrive to do a story on her nintieth birthday.

Photo courtesy of The Newport Plain Talk.

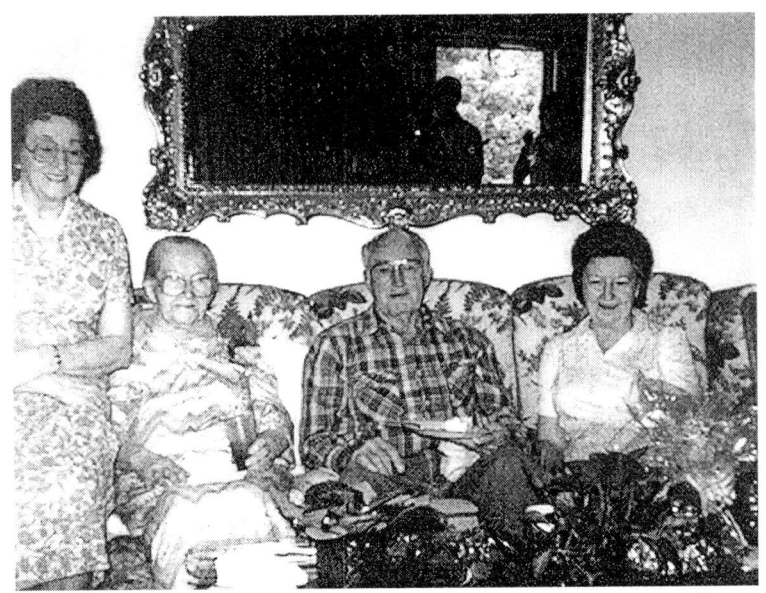

June, Etta, Jack, and Belle pose in Belle's living room during a special occasion to celebrate her 93rd birthday—1990.

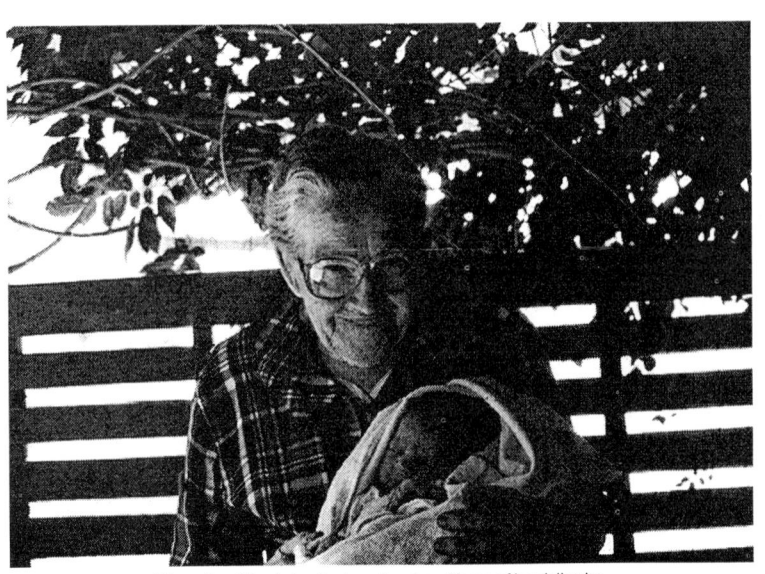

Etta smiles sitting in her front porch swing with one of her deliveries.

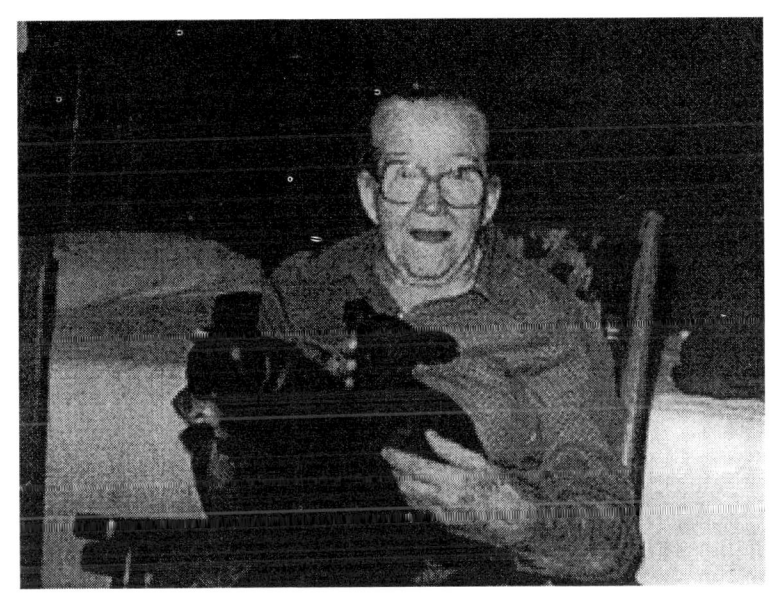

The photographer catches Etta by surprise as she sits in her wooden rocker with her pets, Spider and Little Bit.

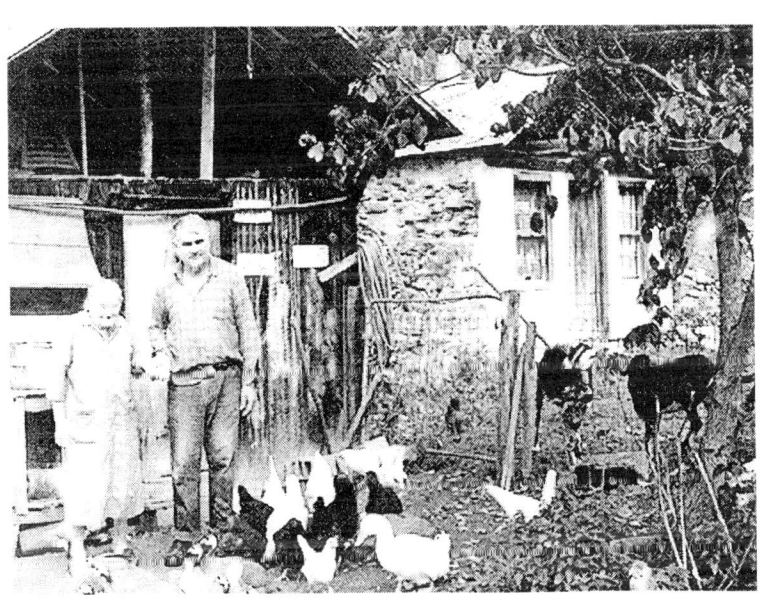

Etta stands in her backyard with a friend as they get ready to feed her many farm animals.

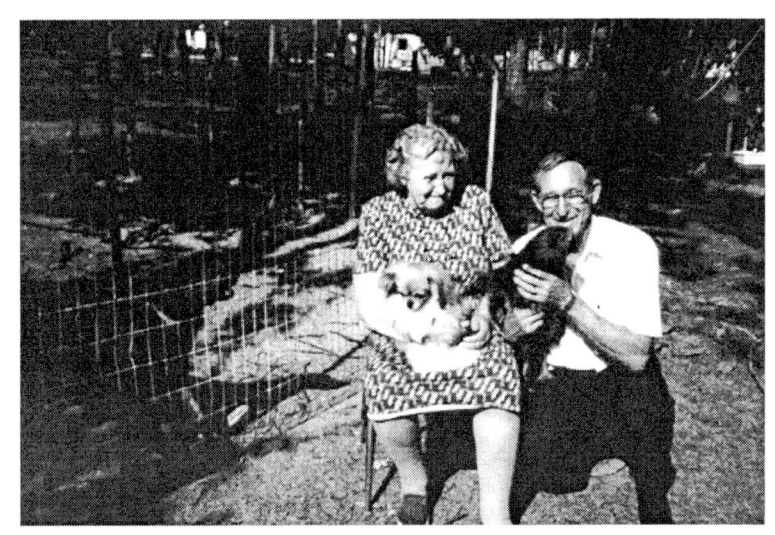

Alverta Taylor and her son, James Taylor, send Etta a picture of her prize rooster at her home in Jacksonville, Florida.

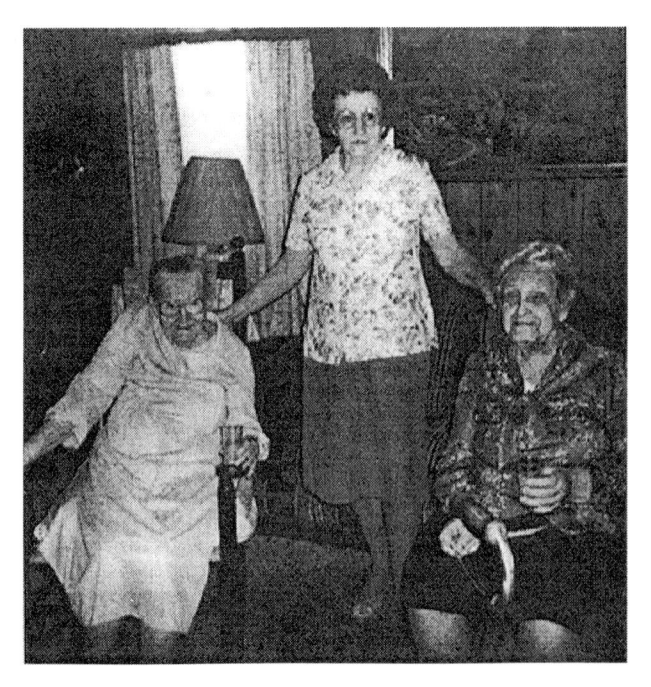

Etta's sister, Alverta, visits her from Jacksonville, Florida, while she is in Tennessee visiting with relatives. Picture taken while Etta was staying with June after her retirement as a midwife.

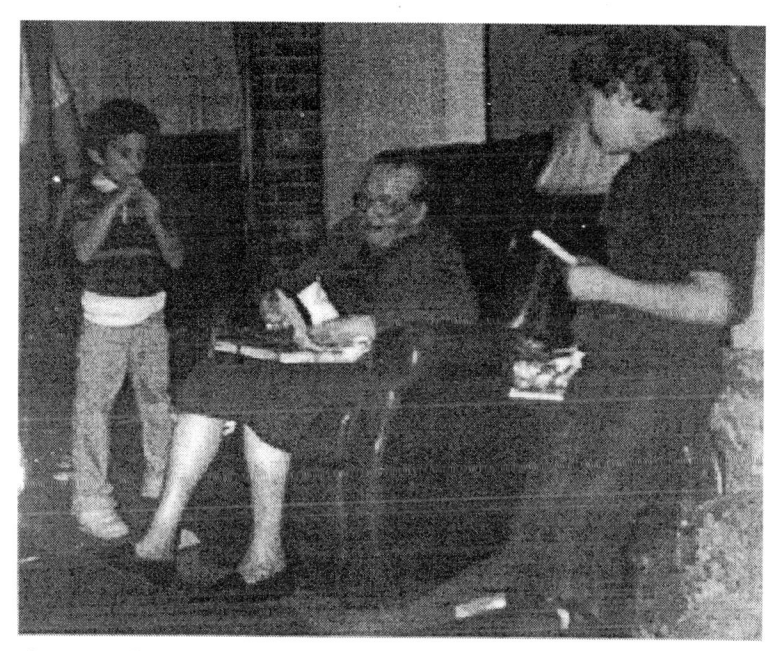

Etta opens her Christmas gifts at Belle's house. Mark Guillot stands on the left, and Russel Smith stands on the right, both great-grandsons of hers.

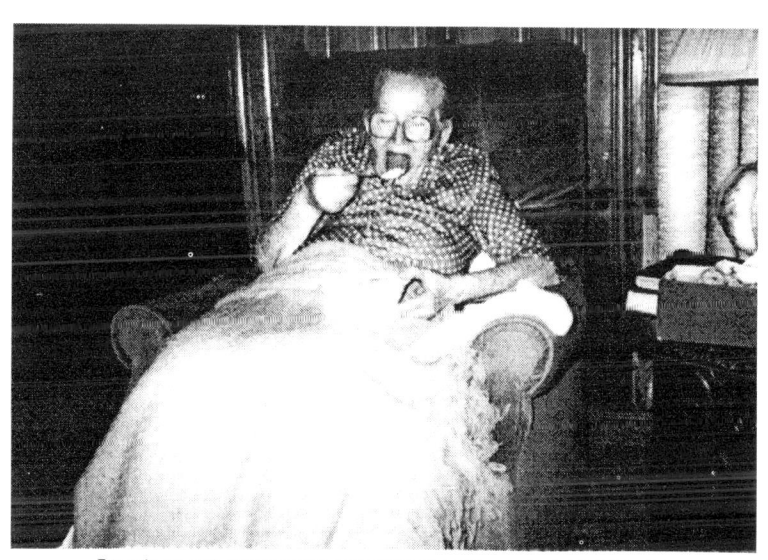

Etta enjoys a cool, refreshing bowl of ice cream as an afternoon treat at Belle's house.

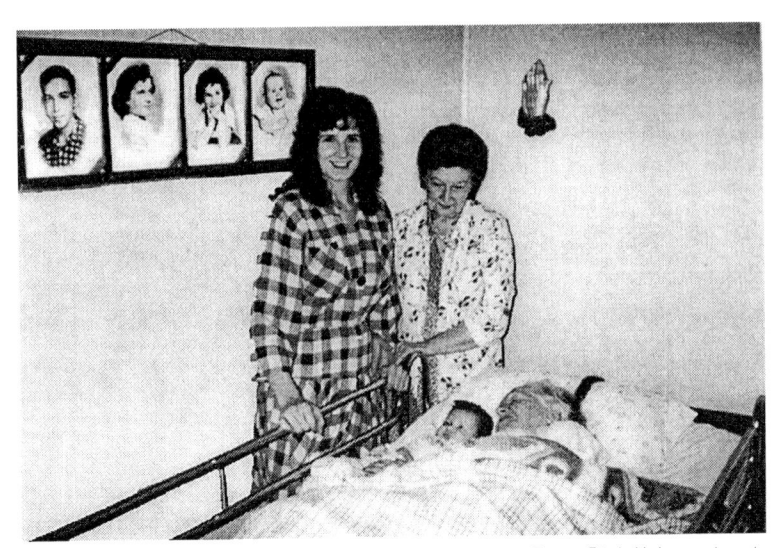

Renina Sparks stands with her grandmother, Belle, and great-grandmother, Etta, as Etta holds her great-great-grandson in the bed with her at Belle's house. Renina is the firstborn child of Lynda and Edd Burgin. Her son is Caleb Sparks.

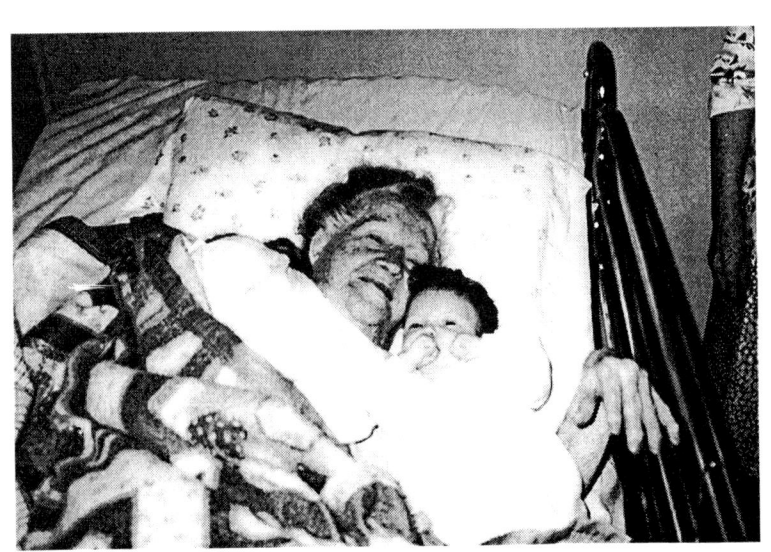

Etta enjoys holding a baby in her arms again as she and Caleb relax in bed. Caleb had been crying for a long while, but as soon as Renina laid him beside Etta he hushed instantly, and did not cry any more. Etta had a special way with babies.

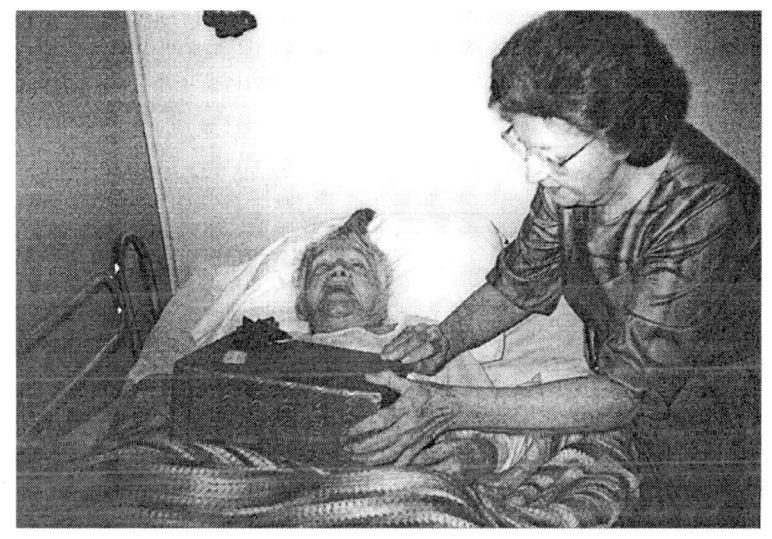

Christmas Day 1993. Belle helps Etta open one of her gifts.

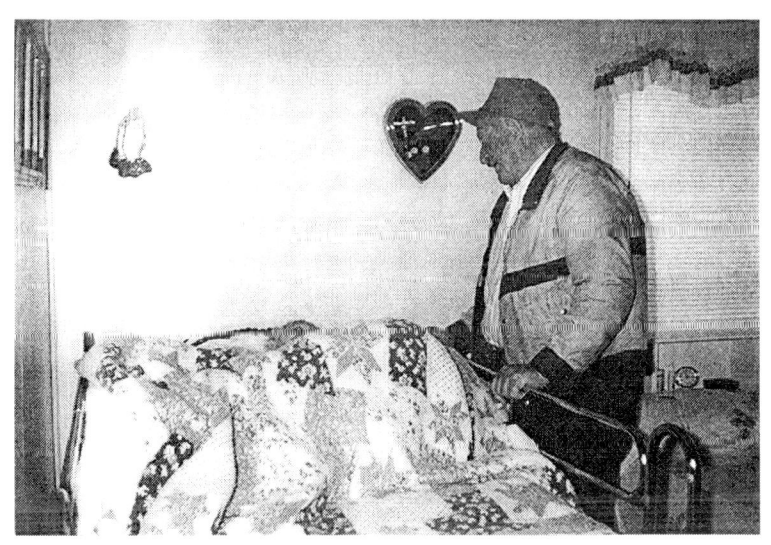

Etta's only living brother, Furman, stops by to visit with Etta—1994.

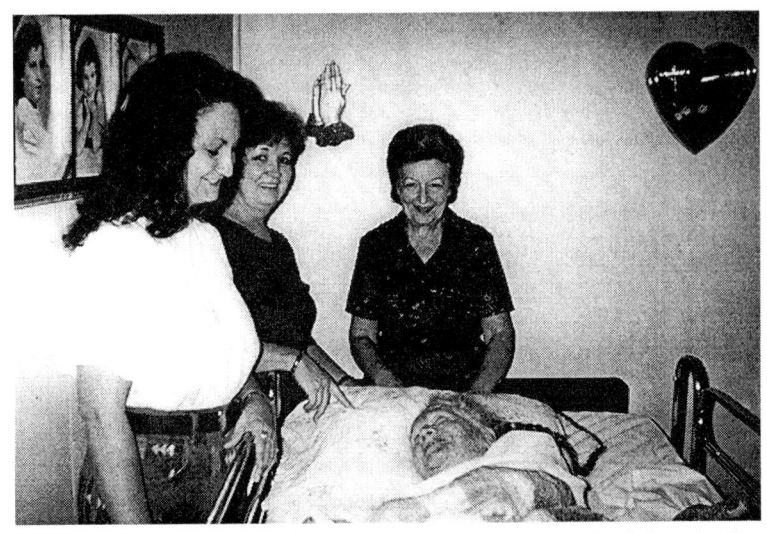

Granddaughters, Debbie Jones, and Valerie Jones Thornton visit with their grandmother. Belle stands at the head of the bed—1994.

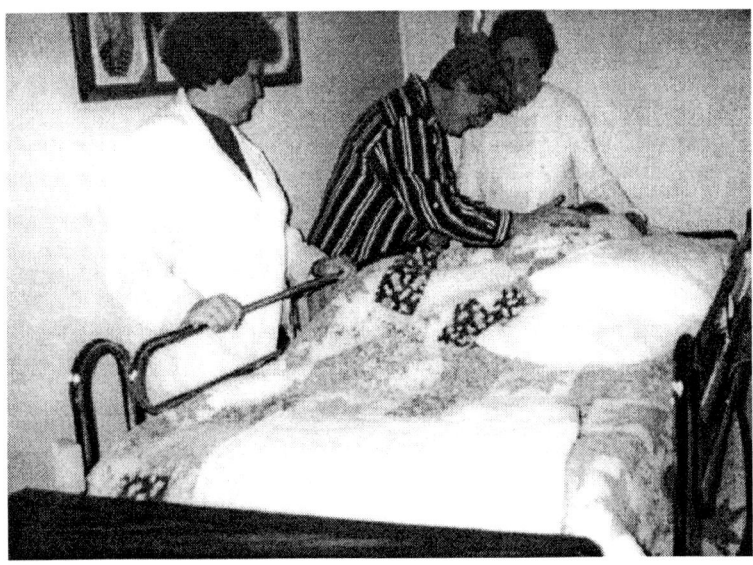

Johnnie Sue stands beside her sister, Virginia Ann Gilliland-Brown as she strokes her grandmother's face affectionately. June stands at the head of the bed.

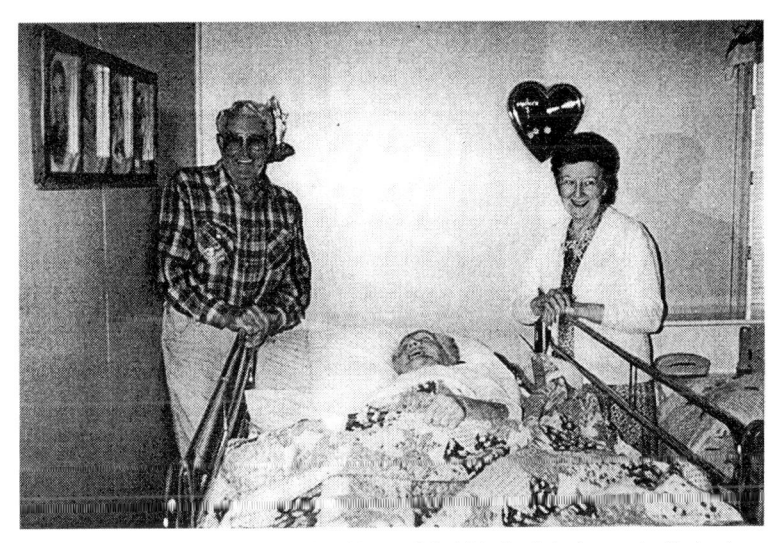

Something amusing has Etta's son, Jack, and daugter, Belle, joining in with her for some healthy, hearty laughter—1994.

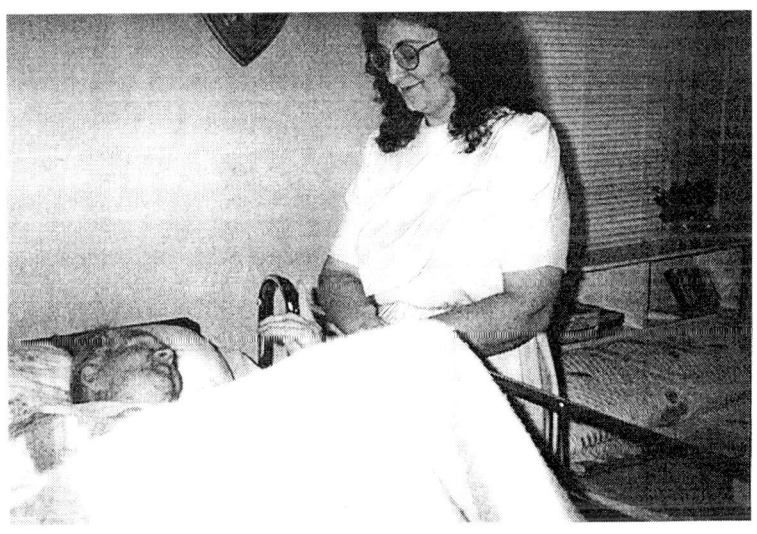

Granddaughter, Venida Pangle, listens to Etta tell many stories of past experiences during her life—1994.

Part V

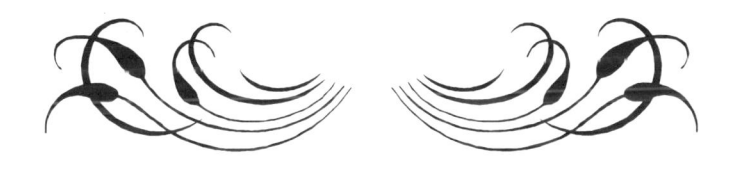

Middle-Aged And Counting

Part V

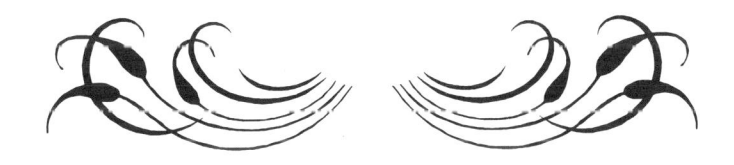

Middle-Aged And Counting

The summer of 1959 brought with it hot, humid temperatures—typical summer weather for East Tennessee. Etta and Harrison had been walking over to Claude and Bonnie Stokely's house for the past week, which was about a three-mile walk, to take food to Claude and Bonnie's daughter, Nellie, who was suffering with rheumatic fever. Harrison always wore long-sleeved shirts under his overalls, even in the summer months. Etta usually never wore sleeves above the elbow. Harrison and Etta wiped the sweat from their brow as they climbed the hills through the woodlands leading to Claude's house. Sometimes Etta lucked out and caught a ride with a neighbor who was going her way; if not, she walked. She wanted to make sure Nellie had medicine and proper nourishment to help her combat her illness. Etta visited the Stokely home every day for over two weeks, bringing food for Nellie, and the girl started to recover. Etta never charged Claude for helping Nellie. Etta was like that with everyone. She was always very giving of herself. She did not have one single selfish bone in her body. She never saw a stranger, or refused to help anyone she could.

On different occasions, Dick and Emily and their children came to visit with Harrison and Etta on the weekend, only to find that John and June were also there with their children. Floyd and Belle and their kids always came over, too, when Belle's sisters were there, and Jack and Juanita would drop in, too. It was like a family reunion on these particular days.

Floyd Ray, Geraldine, Susan and Virginia Ann were all close to the same age, so they hung around together; Jimmy, Sandra and Linda were close to one another's age, so they played together; Darrell and Venida were only about one month apart in age, so they teamed up together; Johnnie Sue and Sharon Kay had only one year's difference in their age, which led them to develop a very close bond with one another. Debbie was still a baby, so she stayed close to her mother.

Etta always cooked a large lunch whenever her children came to visit. She usually always prepared her famous chicken and dumplings, along with vegetables from the garden, homemade loaf bread, cornbread, and of course, buttermilk. She never had to worry about dessert because she always had plenty of fruit pies and vanilla cookies with ice cream on hand to go around for everyone. After the meal, Emily, June, and Belle helped clean the dishes while all the children went out to play. Etta had all kinds of farm animals for the children to enjoy. There were cats, kittens, dogs, ducks, chickens, rabbits, pigeons, guineas, peacocks, and Etta's milk cow, Blossom. It was a real treat for the children when Blossom would have a new calf. Everyone would walk up to the barn in the field behind Etta's house to take a peek at the cute, bug-eyed, furry baby as it struggled to balance itself on its unstable legs. Johnnie Sue and Sharon Kay were most captivated by the kittens which lived in the top of the smokehouse in the backyard. The kittens would come down and play in the yard once they were old enough to climb down. Watching kittens play together can be a delight to one's soul, especially a small child. After playing with the animals, the children would play hide and seek, or tag, or play in the small brook which trickled peacefully at the edge of Etta's front yard. When four o'clock came, everyone was usually ready to return to their own home to get ready for evening church service. Dick and Emily returned to Newport; John and June returned to Morristown, and Floyd and Belle returned to their new house in the Jonestown area of Del Rio, just across a small mountain from where they lived in Smithville.

These family get-togethers were so special to Etta. She loved having her children and grandchildren surrounding her. It instilled a close bond between all her grandchildren as they grew up, and it taught them the importance of having a close, loving family—a lesson they would need to know as they grew up. These would be precious memories they could all look back on, and cherish in their hearts forever.

It was becoming increasingly difficult for Etta to find a ride to her mother's house in London. A lot of times she ended up having to walk there and back. Harrison knew what he had to do. In 1961, at the age of 65, Harrison applied for his Tennessee driver's license in Newport. After passing the test, he bought his first car, a Ford Falcon. A huge burden was lifted from Etta now that she no longer had to intrude on her neighbors to find a ride.

Now that Harrison had his own car, he was often called upon by friends and neighbors for a ride to Del Rio or Newport. He stayed quite busy providing transportation for people in the community. Usually, he only charged his passengers for the gas the trip consumed, but there were many times he never received any payment at all. Harrison still did what he could to help his neighbors. He and Etta were very much alike in that respect; they both enjoyed helping others, payment or no payment.

Harrison arrived at Novie's house each morning around six o'clock. Etta would already have her mother's breakfast over, and have her cleaned up for the day ahead. Etta cleaned the house when she arrived in the evening. When Harrison and Etta arrived back at their house, they went to the barn to milk Blossom. Etta thought as much of her cow as she did any of her farm pets. Blossom seemed to realize Etta's love for her, and she returned it to Etta the only way she could: she produced lots and

Etta "Granny" Nichols—Last of the Old-Timey Midwives

lots of milk, and occasionally she rubbed the top of her head affectionately against Etta's stomach. After the milking was done, Etta always seemed to find something to do to stay busy. When the chores were out of the way, Etta found the time to bake her mother's favorite cookies, the plain vanilla ones. She never used any mix. Etta made everything from scratch in her kitchen. She rolled the dough in her hands and shaped the cookies into neat round forms on the baking sheet. Before long the sweet aroma of Etta's vanilla cookies engulfed the house as they baked in the oven. Ummm...ummm...they tasted so good with a big glass of ice-cold, sweet milk in the evening as a snack! Everyone loved Etta's vanilla cookies, so she always tried to keep some in the big glass cookie jar which sat on her kitchen cupboard. After the evening milking was done, Harrison drove his wife back to Novie's where she stayed until the following morning, then the routine started all over again...unless an expectant mother needed her services. On such occasions, Etta had to get another family member to stay with Novie.

Years passed with Etta following pretty much the same peaceful routine from one day to the next, although there were some days when life could become quite hectic, Etta always managed to remain calm, only showing the gentler side of her spirit.

In August of 1963, Sharon started school at Del Rio Elementary. Her teacher was Mrs. Opal Corn Myers. Everyone in the community called her Miss Opal (Opal was the little girl who, at 11, told Etta about Leonora Whittaker [Christy] and her wonderful work at the Mission School.) Opal's dream of becoming a school teacher had become a reality. She had been teaching in the Cocke County School System for many years, and she made a wonderful teacher.

On March 13, 1964, Datis Cagle pulled into Etta's driveway. His wife Nancy was ready to give birth to their sixth child. Etta had delivered all of the Cagle children. Alberta on March 11, 1952; Charlotte on March 22, 1956; Francis on December 20, 1957; Marvin on March 1, 1960; and Martha Kay on March 10, 1962. All the girls weighed over 10 pounds, and Marvin weighed 12 pounds.

Etta had been with Nancy for a couple of days now, but she had not given birth yet. Etta sat down in the rocking chair and drifted off to sleep during the afternoon. Nancy poked Datis in the side with her elbow, "Look at Granny. Wonder what she's dreamin' about?" Nancy whispered. Etta was scuffling her feet all over the floor. Nancy and Datis laughed quietly as they watched. Etta opened her eyes and saw the two smiling widely. "You was dreamin' something crazy, Granny. Do you remember what it was?" Datis asked.

Etta's expression showed she was in deep thought trying to remember her dream. "Yeah. I remember now what it was. I was in the chicken house and I was movin' the chickens out of my way with my feet," Etta giggled.

On March 16, 1964, Nancy gave birth to another 10-pound baby girl. They named her Patricia. Again, Datis paid Etta $15 and drove her home.

On December 30, 1964, Etta was staying with R. D. and Martha Click to deliver their fourth child. Etta had delivered the previous three children for this couple, also. Their firstborn child was a boy, but he died at birth due to water on his brain, Etta named him Gary Lynn Click. He was born on November 2, 1958. The second child was Joyce Sue, born on September 20, 1959, weighing 9 pounds and 2 ounces. She could not breathe at birth and the valve going to her heart would not close. Joyce Sue had to be taken to a hospital in Knoxville, about a two-hour drive away. The baby survived and became a healthy child. The third child was a boy, Anthony Dean, weighing 6 pounds and 5 ounces. He was born on December 18, 1962.

Nightfall came and everyone was ready to go to bed. Etta crawled into bed with Martha. "Wake me when it's time," Etta told her, then turned over on her side and went to sleep.

Around 1:00 A.M. Martha woke Etta. Her pains were coming quicker and stronger. Etta got up and tended to her patient. At 2:30 A.M. on December 31, 1964, Martha gave birth to a 7-pound baby girl. They named her Angela Dawn. When morning came Etta was paid $15 then she returned home.

In the spring of 1965, Lynda (who had changed the spelling of her name), was staying with Etta while her husband, Edd Burgin, was working in Ohio. Blossom was overdue to give birth to a new calf. After the noon meal was over, and the kitchen was cleaned, Etta looked over at Lynda and said, "Well, Lynda, let's just go up there and get that calf." Etta put on her rubber galoshes, which she always wore to the barn, and her brown, calf-length coat, and the two women walked to the barn to bring a new life into the world. Blossom was lying in the barn outside from her stall. Sixteen-year-old Lynda stood watching in amazement as her grandmother knelt down and pushed her arm up into the cow ever so gently. Lynda listened as Etta talked to Blossom in a kind and gentle tone to help relieve her fear. Lynda had never witnessed anything quite like this before. Etta gripped the baby calf firmly as she withdrew her arm from Blossom's womb. "Here's your baby!" Etta said to Blossom excitedly. It was brown and white like its mother. Blossom licked her baby clean as the new calf took a bug-eyed view of the world around it. "It's another little bull," Etta said disappointedly. "Why couldn't you have been a heifer? I need another milk cow. Blossom is getting old. She won't last many more years. Well, you're a cute little thang no matter what you are." Etta turned and looked at Lynda standing behind her. "The last several calves from Blossom have all been little bulls. We've just had a run of bulls around here," Etta said with a giggle.

The little bull made several attempts to stand on its lanky little legs before it was successful. Lynda laughed as the little bull looked up at her with its front legs spread wide apart in an awkward attempt to balance itself. "Oh, look, Mamaw! It's so cute," Lynda said joyfully.

After getting Blossom and her new baby into the stall, Etta and Lynda started walking back to the house through the frequently traveled path in the field. "I know you're used to this kind of stuff, Mamaw, but this is one of those times I will always remember as being a special occasion I shared with you," Lynda said in a heartwarming tone.

Etta looked at her granddaughter and smiled proudly.

On April 26, 1967, Marvin Turner brought Etta to deliver his and Joann's baby. It was midday when Joann went into labor. "Push with all your strength, Joann," Etta instructed.

Marvin stood beside the bed watching in awe as his wife gave birth. When the baby came out it had the cord wrapped around its neck and had turned blue. Marvin thought the baby was dead and he passed out on the floor right then and there. Etta could not help him because she was too busy working with the baby. Once the cord was off, Etta shook the baby and she started crying. Poor Marvin was still on the floor. Etta reached down and shook him awake once the crisis was over. "You have a 10-pound baby girl up here. Don't you want to get up from there and take a look at your daughter?" Etta laughed.

Marvin was ecstatic. His baby was alive after all! The happy couple named their little girl Angie. Marvin paid Etta her fee of $15, then drove her home after she made sure the baby was okay.

On June 22, 1967, all of Novie's children, grandchildren, and great-grandchildren gathered together at Novie's small three-room house in London to celebrate her 90th birthday. Relatives caught up with the goings-on in one another's life as the children played horseshoes, tag, and red rover-red rover. The weather was hot and humid as the sun beamed down. Waitsel, Etta, Furman, and Willie had a photo taken standing together in front of Novie's house while they were there together.

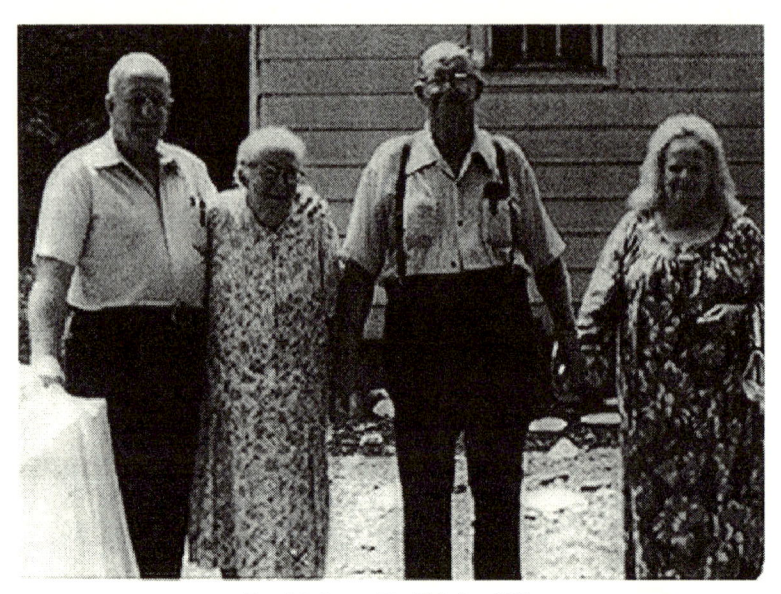

From left: Furman, Etta, Waitsel, and Willie

    Several homemade plywood tables, which were supported by wooden sawhorses underneath, were constructed by the men and placed in Novie's yard and draped with white tablecloths.

    Each woman had prepared a dish to bring to the birthday gathering. After the meal, Novie's birthday cake was brought out. Novie had some help blowing out the candles, then it was sliced and passed around. After everyone was full from the meal and cake, the men relaxed in the front yard telling "fishing stories" and making casual conversation while the women cleaned the dishes from the table.

    Etta hated to see the day come to an end. Even though she lived close to some of her brothers and sisters, she rarely had a chance to visit with them, and with Alvertie and Willie living so far away, she did not know how long it would be before she would see them again. But the time did come when everyone had to say their good-byes and return to their homes, leaving a certain sadness in Etta's heart. She felt this would be the last time the family would all be gathered together to celebrate their mother's birthday, but she hoped she was wrong.

Two or three weeks after Novie's birthday party, Etta had to move her mother in with her.

Novie had taken ill and needed constant supervision. Novie did not put up a fuss this time, maybe she just did not have the strength. A few weeks later, Harrison's mother also became ill, and Etta took her in to care for as well.

Since Etta could no longer leave home for any length of time, she arranged to have the bedroom behind the kitchen to be made into a "baby room." The women would have to come to her to give birth now. She placed two twin-size beds in the room, and had a sink and commode installed in one corner for her patients. State health officials donated an incubator for Etta to use with premature babies weighing less than 5 1/2 pounds. She would place the infant in it until assistance from the Valentine-Shults Hospital in Newport arrived. She placed the incubator between the two beds next to the wall. Her baby scales, which she purchased by trading in her S&H green stamps, was placed on a small table at the other side of the room. Everything was now ready for Etta to begin using her new birthing room. Etta awaited her first in-home patient.

• • • • • •

In the summer of 1967 Etta made a routine visit to Dr. Muncy at his office in Jefferson City. Dr. Muncy performed a breast examination during Etta's visit and found a lump in her right breast. After doing the regular test to determine if the lump was malignant, the results came back positive. Etta had breast cancer. Dr. Muncy made Etta an appointment with Dr. Zerkle at Saint Mary's in Knoxville for the following day. Dr. Zerkle would have to perform exploratory surgery to determine if the cancer had spread to the point where Etta would need to have a mastectomy. Harrison drove Etta back to Del Rio from Jefferson City. She packed some clothes and made arrangements for a neighbor to stay and help with her mother and mother-in-law, then Harrison drove her to Saint Mary's Hospital in Knoxville. Of course Etta was upset by the formidable news Dr. Muncy revealed to her, but she did not want to worry her children, so she never told them what the doctor had found, or that she was scheduled for surgery the next day. After seeing Etta checked into her room at the hospital, Harrison had to return home to take care of the evening milking. He wanted to stay with Etta, but certain chores had to be tended to. The following day Belle found out from her father that Etta was scheduled for surgery that morning. Belle immediately called June, Jack, and Emily to tell them the shocking news. Neither Emily nor Jack could leave home that particular morning, but June and Belle arranged to meet one another in Morristown and head to Knoxville as fast as they could. The women were upset that their mother had tried to keep them in the dark about her surgery. June and Belle arrived at the hospital just as the nurses had wheeled

Etta into the operating room. Etta never knew they were there.

The clock seemed to tick slower than usual as June and Belle waited for some news from the doctor. Finally, after several hours, Dr. Zerkle came out to inform them that the cancer had spread too far to save Etta's right breast. He'd had to perform the mastectomy, but he felt confident he had gotten all the cancer. June and Belle were very disturbed by the news the doctor revealed to them, but relieved to know the cancer was gone.

When Etta woke up, her two daughters were standing beside her bed to give her all the emotional support they could. June and Belle both stayed two nights at the hospital until Etta was released to go home. Within two weeks of her surgery Etta was out hanging clothes on the line. Etta seemed to be coping quite well on the surface with her mastectomy, but for a woman to have her breast removed is an ordeal that takes a tremendous amount of inner strength.

• • • • • •

Novie's health steadily deteriorated. On November 22, 1967, Novie took her last breath at the age of 90. The funeral services were held in Etta's house with Rev. Colwell performing the eulogy. Etta's small four-room house was packed with friends and relatives attending the service. Etta's children tried to comfort her, but once again Etta had to turn to God for strength to say good-bye to her dearly beloved mother. Nova Melinda Jane Turner Grigsby was laid to rest in the Jonestown Cemetery on Highway 107 in Del Rio.

After Novie's death, Etta never could bring herself to bake vanilla cookies again. They were her mother's favorite, and she found it too painful, even though everyone else loved them, too.

On different occasions Etta's grandchildren would come to spend the weekend with her, especially Venida and Sharon since they lived so close to her. One weekend Sharon arrived on Friday evening. When darkness fell, it was bedtime, usually between eight and nine o'clock. Sharon was not used to going to bed so early, but since her grandmother had no television there really was not anything else to do. Harrison took the skeleton key to wind up the wooden Ingram clock which sat on top of the fireplace mantel then retired to the bedroom. Sharon would sleep with Etta in the full-size bed in one corner of the living room. Even though Sharon was not sleepy, the rhythm of the tick tock from the clock soon put her to sleep.

Five o'clock came with a loud chime from the clock. Etta and Harrison got up and got dressed. Etta proceeded to the kitchen to cook breakfast while Harrison went outside to open the chicken coop and feed the animals. Sharon was used to sleeping late on Saturday mornings, but had no such luck at Grandma's house. Sharon walked into the kitchen still trying to wake-up. Etta handed her a large bowl and asked if she wanted to gather the eggs from the henhouse. "Pick'em up and put'em in the bowl real easy so they won't crack," Etta told her.

Once inside the hen house Sharon went around to each nest gathering the eggs. One hen still remained on its nest and was giving Sharon a malevolent look. Sharon was afraid to get too close to the hen—she had seen Etta's hens and roosters flog people before. Just then the hen let out a loud cackle and flew from its nest to the ground, running outside. Sharon about had a heart attack. The bird had just missed her head! Sharon quickly gathered the eggs from the last nest and took them to Etta. Etta washed the eggs and placed them in egg crates to sell to her customers for 25 cents per dozen. She sold milk, which she poured into half-gallon glass jars for $1.00 per gallon, and her homemade butter brought 50 cents per pound. If people were not coming to her house for medicine, or to have a baby, they came for her eggs, milk, or butter.

Saturday was filled with people coming and going to buy this, or that, or maybe just to "sit and visit a spell." After Etta cleaned the supper dishes it was time to do the evening milking. Sharon followed her grandmother to the barn through the trail in the field. "Do you want to see if you can milk?" Etta asked Sharon.

Sharon was excited. "Yeah, if you'll show me how."

Etta hollered at Blossom, who was grazing in the field, to come on and get milked. Blossom obeyed and started walking toward the barn. Sharon stood outside the barn as Etta went to the storage room where she kept the cow's grain. Blossom must have known something was up. She walked into the barn and stood looking Sharon in the eye, then all of a sudden Blossom ran toward Sharon and butted her, knocking her down right beside a big pile of manure.

Sharon almost lost her breath, but the only thing hurt was her pride. Etta came around the corner about that time and saw Sharon on the ground. Sharon explained what had happened. Etta scolded Blossom and whipped her on the rear with a rope. Blossom went into the milking stall without hesitation. Etta poured the grain into the feed bin then pulled up her short milking stool. "Take a seat right here," Etta instructed Sharon. "Now put your hand around the tit at the top and pull down as you squeeze."

Sharon made several attempts before she finally got any milk to come out. Once she understood the technique of milking, the next thing was to master the art of hitting the bucket with the milk instead of the ground!

After the chores were done and it was dark, Etta let down her hair, which she always wore in a twisted bun on the back of her head, and let Sharon brush it out for her. "Have you ever had your hair cut, Mamaw?" Sharon asked as she stroked the brush down Etta's back.

"No, I never have. There was one time I almost cut it when I was younger, but just as I put the scissors up to it a voice spoke to me and told me not to do it. 'A woman's hair is her glory,' the voice told me. So I never did even think of cutting it after that." It was apparent Etta was telling the truth. Her hair came down past her hips when she let it down.

Sharon continued brushing until she almost put Etta to sleep. Etta twisted her hair around into one strand then put a rubber band around it before going to bed.

Sunday morning came, and once again Sharon had to get up early to attend church services with her grandparents. She took her clothes out to the building Etta called the "wash house," which had a shower in one corner, a washer, and a well pump all occupying the building. After Sharon took a shower, she got dressed for church.

Harrison and Etta were attending church at Fugate Baptist located on the River Road in Del Rio. Sharon enjoyed going to church there. The preacher would get excited and shout praises to God, as members of the congregation shouted "Hallelujah!" The spirit of God was definitely present in that church. After church services, Harrison drove Etta and Sharon home. The rest of the day was spent relaxing on the couch listening to gospel singing on Harrison's radio, which was almost as tall as Sharon, and about three feet wide, while Etta sat on the couch reading the Holy Bible. Harrison occasionally leaned over his brown padded rocking chair to spit tobacco juice into the spittoon sitting on the floor beside him. After reading every page in the Sunday newspaper, Harrison picked up his Holy Bible and read it until time to go back for evening church services.

On June 19, 1968, Etta received a knock on her door at 6 A.M. She had just gotten out of bed and was starting breakfast. Etta answered the door to find Melissa Marvene Turner. Melissa was in strong labor. Etta led her to the "baby room" and showed her where to lie down. Betty Burgin occupied the other bed in the room. She had come a day or so before, to give birth. At 8:30 A.M. Melissa gave birth to a whopping 11-pound baby. "I had my last baby in the hospital, and I had a harder time there than I had here. You are just a super lady, Granny," Melissa told

Etta. Melissa stayed until noon, paid Etta $15, then went home. A lot of the women that came to Etta left a few hours after giving birth. They said it was just so much easier on them at Etta's house than what they experienced in the hospital, that they did not need to stay longer.

• • • • • •

On February 24, 1970, Harrison lost his mother. Her health had been slowly deteriorating due to old age. The funeral service was held at Harrison and Etta's house, and she was laid to rest in the Crowder Cemetery on South Highway 107 in Del Rio.

In March of 1970, Dora Stokley knocked on Etta's door at 4 A.M. She gave birth three hours later to a little girl, weighing 9 pounds and 2 ounces, and named her, Lisa. There was another woman in the other bed beside Dora. Dora told her, "This is my second baby. Granny delivered my first'n, too. That time the Del Rio bridge was out, and we had to drive all the way around the River Road to get here. I was afraid I wasn't goin' ta make it in time. That was in May of 1969. That'n was an eight pound, 6 ounce boy. We named him Arnold Jay Stokley. This is changin' the subject, but has Granny fixed any of her biscuits since you've been here? She makes the best biscuits I've ever ate. She don't roll 'em out and use a cutter, she puts the dough all together kind'a thin in the pan and bakes the whole pan like that. Talk about good, nobody can beat her biscuits!"

Etta came in just then to check on the new mother and baby, and to tell them she had been called in an emergency and had to leave for awhile. The women assured Etta they were both okay and would not need her to stay. Several hours later Etta returned. She went in to tell the women she was home. "I've seen a lot of strange things in my lifetime, but what I just witnessed has to take the cake. When I walked into the house where I went to, this girl was on the couch already havin' the baby—I got there just in time. But the funny part is, she didn't even know she was pregnant! She didn't have one stitch of clothes for that baby to put on, so I told her I kept a few baby clothes here at home for my patients, and I'd send Harrison back over there with them until she could buy her some."

"What! She didn't know she was pregnant! Well, I guess she got a surprise, huh?!" Dora laughed. The women talked for a few more minutes then Dora informed Etta, "I believe I feel like goin' on home, Granny. Thank you for takin' such good care of me and the baby. You're such a sweet lady." Four hours after giving birth Dora got up, paid Etta her $15 fee, then Geneva Stokley and Imogene Daniels drove her home.

Later that year Harrison was admitted to Baptist Hospital in Knoxville where Dr. Zerkle would be performing a hemorrhoidectomy on him. Belle took her father a pair of pajamas then returned home. Although this was a painful procedure, it was not serious. Harrison did not need anyone to stay with him during his hospital confinement. When Harrison returned home a couple of days later, he walked into the kitchen where Lynda and Etta stood, and kissed Etta on the lips. "I thought your Granny was the purrtiest woman I ever saw first time I laid eyes on 'er, and I still think she's the purttiest," Harrison told Lynda.

Etta's face turned blood-red from embarrassment. No one had ever seen the couple kiss on the mouth before, only a peck on the cheek. "Not in front of the grandchildren, Harrison," Etta scolded.

Lynda got tickled at Etta. After all, she was now 20 years old and had a child of her own. "It's good to have you back home, Papaw," Lynda said as she walked into the living room. "I'll go in here so you two love birds can be alone," Lynda laughed.

Etta's life as a midwife was becoming more popular around many surrounding counties during this time. Midwives were almost non-existent, which made Etta's life very interesting to more and more people. On July 23, 1970, the following article appeared in The Newport Plain Talk:

Etta "Granny" Nichols—Last of the Old-Timey Midwives

Cocke County Mid-Wife

By Edwina Prisk
Plain Talk Staff Writer

A good number of the babies in the area surrounding Cocke County born in the past half century have not been delivered by a licensed doctor. At least, 1026 babies that we know about have been born with only the presence of a mid-wife. That mid-wife is Mrs. James Harrison Nichols.

Doctor or Granny Nichols, as she is known by many of her patients, is the wife of James Harrison Nichols and they live on the Laurel Branch Road above Nough in the Del Rio section of Cocke County. Mrs. Nichols has lived in that community since she was born.

PRACTICAL EDUCATION

Although Mrs. Nichols has only a grammar school education she has received years of practical knowledge. Both her grandfather, John B. Grisby, and her father, J.L. Grisby, were practicing physicians. She said of her grandfather and father, "They were just country doctors but were said to be the best in this part of the country." Her grandfather practiced for about 10 years and her father for about 30 years. It was not strange or unusual for Mrs. Nichols to accompany her father on his calls and assist him in his work. At times she also accompanied the late Dr. R.W. Smith on some of his calls.

YEARS OF SERVICE

Mrs. Nichols has been bringing babies into this world for the past 40 years and she is still very active. In fact, the last baby she delivered was on Sun-

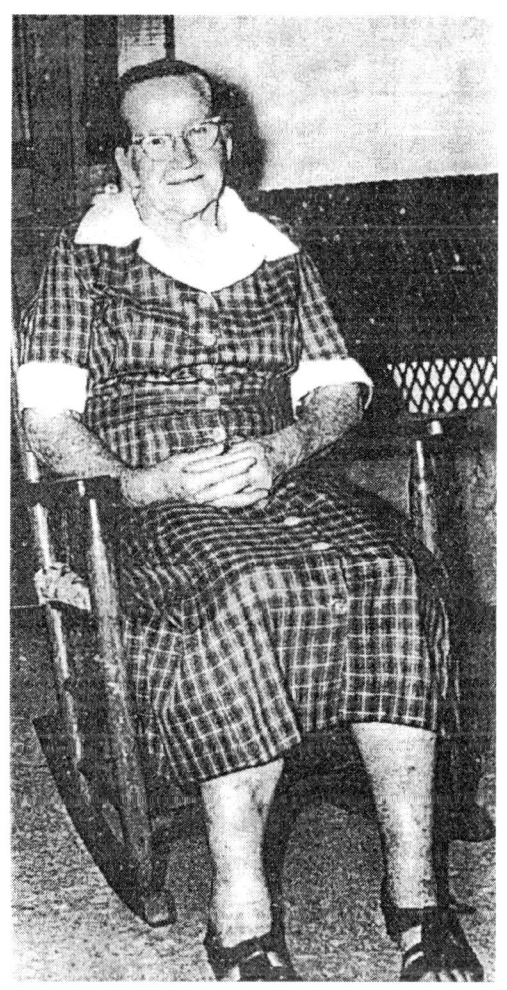

Mrs. James Harrison Nichols

day, June 38, 1970 for Mrs. Barbara Dennis of Bat Harbor.

Mrs. Nichol's vocation was started more or less for her. One day, a neighbor, Mrs. Edtha Morrow, who was about to give birth, called for her father, Dr Grisby. He was not at home and they did not know where he could be found. Asked by the family to come, she checked and delivered her first baby. This was the start.

TRANSPORTATION

During the earlier years Mrs. Nichols went to the home of her patients. She has walked and gone by horseback but usually some member of the family will come for her by car.

TREATMENT

For the past three years she has been delivering the babies in her own home. Because of a family obligation she has not been able to go to the homes of her patients. Therefore, a room was prepared where the patient could come to her. Here the patient can stay until they feel ready to return to their own home. The first baby delivered at her home was on July 17, 1967.

Her patients do not have the help of an anesthetic. Birth is by natural childbirth and an occasional whiff of ether.

Many times the women will come to Mrs. Nichols before the birth of their child to be checked, for instructions, advice, to make arrangements for delivery, or just to talk. However, many times Mrs. Nichols does not know she is going to be asked to deliver a baby until the patient arrives at her home.

HER FAMILY

Mrs. Nichols has a family of her own. She and Mr. Nichols have four children, Emily, June, Jack and Belle, 13 grandchildren and nine great-grandchildren. She has delivered five of her grandchildren and three of her great-grandchildren.

RECORD

The largest baby she has delivered charted 13 pounds on a 25 pound scale. The mother was Mrs. Joe Raines.

The smallest baby to live was one that weighed three and a half pounds, born to Mrs. Carl Hensley.

Mrs. Dan Roberts was her oldest mother at 47 years.

She has delivered two Negro children, thirteen sets of twins, and nine children each to the families of Mrs. Charlie Barrett and Mrs. James Ellison.

She can boast of the fact that she has never lost a mother.

Last year she delivered 30 babies.

She has delivered babies from all communities in Cocke County, Greene-ville, Kodak, Chestnut Hill, Spring Creek and Marshall, N.C. and all of her babies are recorded and registered with the Department of Vital Statistics in Nashville.

UNUSUAL

The most unusual case she can remember happened about a year ago. Mrs. Nichols told this story. "One evening I heard a car pull up and the husband of a patient jumped out. His wife was with him so I started back through the house to get the bed ready for the patient. Before I reached the backroom he came in and said, 'Quick, Mrs. Nichols, the baby is on its way.' I only had time to quickly wash my hands and go to the car. There I delivered an eight pound girl."

HIGH PRAISE

The mothers we have talked with have nothing but high praise for Mrs. Nichols.

Mrs. Nichols delivered five children for Mr. and Mrs. Jack Busler of 804 Cosby Road. Unlike many of Mrs. Nichol's patients the Buslers did not know her until the time came for the delivery. Mrs. Busler said, "My husband went for another mid-wife and came back with Mrs. Nichols. We have used her ever since." All of the Busler babies have been delivered at their home except the youngest, Penny, who was born at the home of Mrs. Nichols. Donnie weighed ten pounds and all the rest of them weighed eight pounds. Mrs. Busler said, "I never went to another doctor except one time when I was having a lot of trouble with my feet swelling. I think I got along just as well with Mrs. Nichols as I could have in the hospital. I really love that woman. She has really been good to me."

The people of Sarah Hester have known Mrs. Nichols all of their lives. Mrs. Nichols was used by her mother, Mrs. Rachel Shelton. Mrs. Hester had her daughter at the home of her mother in Newport. She said, "I am proud to have had Mrs. Nichols as my doctor."

Mr. and Mrs. Datis Cagle lived next door to Mrs. Nichols after they were married. She delivered all of her children at the Cagle home in Cosby. Mrs. Cagle said, "I don't think I could have had any better doctor than Mrs. Nichols. She is a wonderful person and we love her very much." Mrs. Cagle visited Mrs. Nichols several times before the birth of her children to have a checkup, she has never been in a hospital, and all of her babies weighed over ten pounds.

Mr. and Mrs. Hobart Shelton have two fine young sons that were delivered by Mrs. Nichols. Mrs. Shelton lived in the Del Rio Community most of her life and met Mrs. Nichols after she was married. The Sheltons now live at 914 First Street, Newport. She said "Mr. and Mrs. Nichols are such lovely, friendly people. They are good Christian people. Mrs. Nichols is ready to wait on people day or night. My hus-

Etta "Granny" Nichols—Last of the Old-Timey Midwives

And Her Children

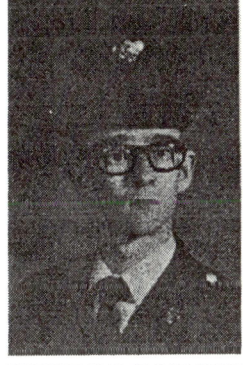

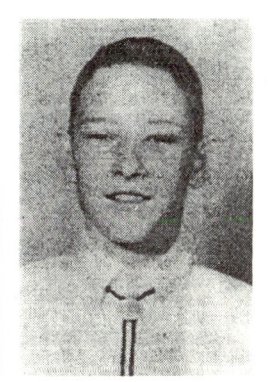

band and I really enjoy being with Mr. and Mrs. Nichols."

GETTING OLDER

Mrs. Nichols is getting along in years but she is still spry enough to have many years left helping women at the most wonderful time in their lives, bringing new life into the world.

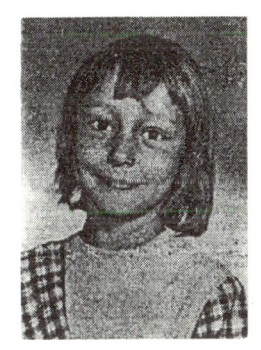

ALMA JEAN HESTER, seven-year old daughter of Mrs. Sarah Hester is another one of the children delivered by Mrs. Nichols.

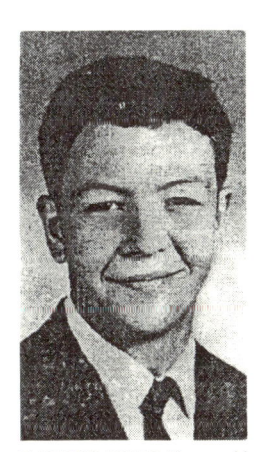

DARRELL JONES, 16-year old son of Mr. and Mrs. Richard Jones was delivered by his grandmother, Mrs. Nichols. Mrs. Jones is the oldest daughter of Mrs. Nichols.

EUGENE AND OLSON SHELTON sons of Mrs. Hobart Shelton, were also delivered by Mrs. Nichols. Eugene left is 20 years of age and is in the Army sttioned in Germany, Olson, 18, is working in Hyattsville, Maryland.

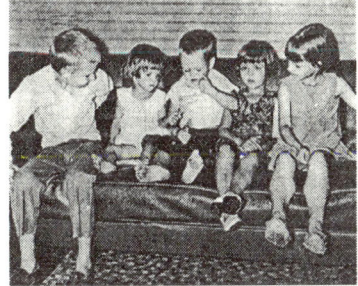

LITTLE BUSLERS—The five children of Mr. and Mrs. Jack Busler, 804 Cosby Road, were delivered by Mrs. Nichols. They are (l. to r.) Jack, 8, Penny Sue, 1, Donnie, 3, Mary 5, and Norma Jean, 7.

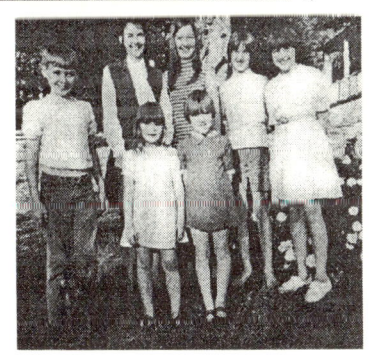

SEVEN IN ONE FAMILY—Seven children of Mr. and Mrs. Datis Cagle were delivered by Mrs. Nichols. They are Marvin, 10, Patricia, 6, Martha, 8, Albertia, 18, Carolyn, 16, Charlotte, 14, and Frances, 11. The Cagles live on Cosby. Their grandparents are Mr. and Mrs. James Ball of Sevierville and Mr. and Mrs. Robert Cagle of Del Rio.

News article and photos courtesy of The Newport Plain Talk.

In July of 1970, Floyd Ray, Belle's son, received orders to go to Vietnam from where he was stationed in Fort Benning, Georgia. Floyd Ray had received his military occupational specialty in the infantry. During his tour in Vietnam, Floyd Ray would be reassigned to the survey platoon, serving with the 101st Airborne Division. His duties would be to establish known survey points for use by the artillery batteries on mountaintop fire bases. This was definitely a dangerous assignment. Floyd Ray was given a one-month leave to go home before his departure for Vietnam.

The weeks flew by at home for Floyd Ray until the time came to leave. During Floyd Ray's last visit with his grandparents, Etta hugged her grandson tight and cried as he turned and walked off her front porch. Would she ever see her oldest grandson alive again?

"See ya later, Poy," Floyd Ray said as he waved to Harrison from the car. Then he was gone.

The next morning, on September 13, 1970, Floyd Ray arose early to head out for the airport in Knoxville. As Belle walked past Floyd Ray's bedroom she noticed him standing there looking around the room as if he might be wondering if this would be the last time he would see it. Belle walked back into the living room to give her son some time alone. Later, Floyd Ray said an emotional good-bye to his mother. His sisters were still in bed. Lynda had come over to spend the night so she could visit with her brother before his departure that morning. Lynda heard her brother leaving as she lay in her bed, but could not bring herself to say good-bye. Lynda waited until she knew Floyd Ray was outside then she went into the bathroom and watched through tear-stained eyes as her brother disappeared around the curve below the house. Floyd Ray did not want the family to go with him to the airport; he wanted to remember his family as they were at home, so Floyd drove his son to McGee Tyson Airport in Knoxville alone. From there he would be departing for Fort Lewis, Washington for two weeks before leaving to go on to Vietnam.

Floyd shook his son's hand and patted him on the back. "Keep your head down, and come back to us alive," Floyd said through teary eyes.

"That's my plan," Floyd Ray answered with a smile, as he picked up his bags, then disappeared through the gate.

Floyd watched the plane take off that carried his son away from the safety of home. He remembered serving in World War II himself, and knew the dangers his only son would be facing. Floyd waved through the airport windows, hoping his son could see him. Tears streamed down his cheeks as the plane disappeared into the clouds. Floyd Ray was gone, but he would remain in the prayers of the family.

• • • • • •

On January 23, 1971, Dick and Emily had just finished breakfast when Emily began to complain with a terrible headache. "I believe I'll go in here and lie down on the couch awhile and see if my head will stop hurting," Emily told Dick.

Dick and his son, Darrell, worked on their dairy farm not too far from the house. "I'll come back in to check on you in a little while," Dick answered. When Dick came back, Emily was still lying on the couch. "How are you feeling?" Dick asked.

"I believe I'm feeling a little better," Emily answered. "You go on back to work. I'll be fine."

Later Dick came in once more to check on his wife. This time she lay unconscious on the couch. Dick shook her gently trying to get her to wake up. No response came from Emily. Dick ran to the door and hollered for Darrell. Darrell knew something was terribly wrong from his father's tone. "Darrell, go next door and get help." Before Darrell went for help he ran into the kitchen and got a spoon to put in his mother's mouth so she would not swallow her tongue. Soon Darrell and the nurse who lived close by came running through the front door. "Call an ambulance!" the woman yelled. She gave Emily mouth-to-mouth resuscitation until the ambulance arrived. Dick rode up front in the ambulance as Emily was taken to Morristown-Hamblen Hospital. The doctor said Emily had suffered a light stroke.

The next day Emily developed pneumonia and her condition worsened. After spending three days at Morristown-Hamblen Hospital the family decided to move Emily to Baptist Hospital in Knoxville. Again Dick rode in front of the ambulance while Valerie and Etta rode in the back with Emily. Etta never left her daughter during her hospital stay as she fasted and prayed for nine days straight.

On February 2, the doctors seemed to think Emily's health was improving somewhat so they allowed the fam-

Etta "Granny" Nichols—Last of the Old-Timey Midwives

ily to visit with her for five minutes, one person at a time. All of Emily's family was there, except her 11-year-old daughter, Debbie, who was staying with friends during her mother's illness, and Jack and Harrison. Etta asked someone to call Jack and get him to drive Harrison down now that Emily could have visitors. June and Belle were already there. Valerie and her husband decided to go to the cafeteria to eat after Valerie had her turn visiting with her mother. When Etta's turn came to see Emily she went in and stood over her daughter's bed and took her hand, rubbing it gently. Just then Emily went into convulsions. Etta screamed for help and soon the room was filled with hospital staff. As family members waited outside the room they could hear Emily fighting for her life. Then quietness. The doctor came out and led the family to the chapel. "I'm afraid Mrs. Jones has died from an aneurysm in her brain. I'm so sorry," the doctor informed them.

Tears filled the eyes and hearts of all the family members as they tried to absorb the horrible news. As Valerie and Bunton returned from the cafeteria, they noticed everyone was in the chapel...Valerie knew her mother was gone.

When Jack arrived with Harrison, Etta met him in the hallway. Etta looked up at her husband through her tears and told him, "Emily's gone. She died." Harrison was shocked. "Oh, she did?" he answered in disbelief. They joined the rest of the family back in the chapel and grieved together.

Later that day when Etta and Harrison returned home, friends and neighbors brought food and offered their sympathy. Losing her daughter was the worst thing Etta had ever experienced. Although Etta always grieved quietly, it was apparent her heart had been shattered from her loss.

The funeral was held at Westside Funeral Home in Morristown two days later. Emily Laura Nichols Jones was laid to rest in the Jarnigan Cemetery, also in Morristown.

After the funeral services Harrison and Etta returned home. Lynda went to be with her grandmother to try and comfort her. When Lynda walked in the front door, Etta was sitting on the couch looking out the side window, as tears streamed down her face. Etta looked up at Lynda and spoke in a cracked voice, "I didn't ever think one of my children would go before me." Etta leaned over and put her face in her hands and sobbed.

Part VI

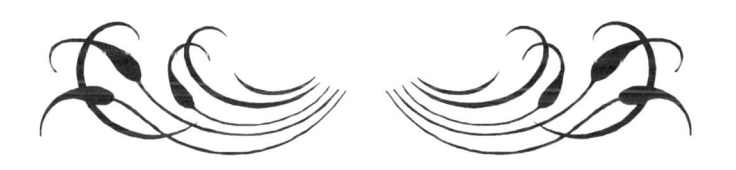

Becoming A Living Legend

Part VI

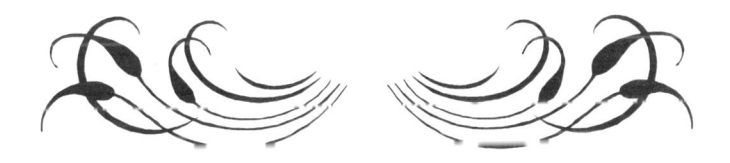

Becoming A Living Legend

*F*loyd Ray served 11 months and 3 weeks in Vietnam. On September 11, 1971, Floyd Ray received his Honorable Discharge from the United States Army, ranking Sergeant E-5. Floyd Ray had survived numerous close calls from enemy artillery fire. Now, at last, he could

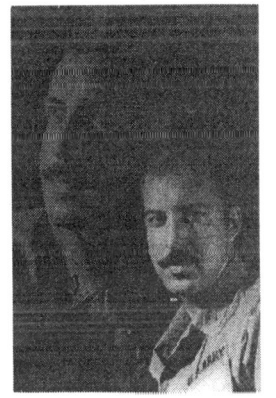

Sergeant Floyd R. Smith

leave the death and devastation of the Vietnam War behind and return home to his family.

Floyd, Belle, Etta, Lynda, Venida, and Sharon waited anxiously at the McGee Tyson airport in Knoxville for Floyd Ray's plane to land. John and June also came to welcome Floyd Ray home. Floyd Ray had always been close to them. June and Etta were sitting in chairs with their backs turned to the gate where Floyd Ray would be entering the building, while Belle sat facing the entrance. When Belle saw her son she jumped up and was about to tell the others he was there, but Floyd Ray put his finger to his mouth to signal his mother to be quiet. Floyd Ray walked up behind his grandmother and gently placed his hand on her shoulder. Etta looked up to find Floyd Ray standing there. She sprang from her seat and raised her hands up to God, and shouted. "Thank you, Jesus!" as tears of joy flowed down her cheeks. "My, my, don't you look a sight for sore eyes!" Etta continued as she wrapped her arms around Floyd Ray.

Floyd Ray laughed and replied, "So do you, Mamaw—so do all of you."

Belle looked at her firstborn child and realized the son she had always thought of as her little boy was now truly a responsible, mature young man. Floyd's heart filled with pride when he watched his son walk proudly in uniform through the crowd of people in the airport. It thrilled Lynda, Venida, and Sharon to see their older brother again, and know he had returned home safe. After talking with John and June for awhile, Floyd Ray walked from the airport with one arm around Lynda and the other arm around Venida and Sharon as he joked and laughed. It was clear

Floyd Ray was happy to be back with his family. Floyd Ray loaded his luggage in the trunk of Floyd's car, then everyone took their seats in the car and began the journey home. Etta sat in the front seat with Floyd and Belle, while Floyd Ray sat in the back with his sisters. Much talk went on between the family members as Floyd Ray caught up with what was happening on the home front. It was such a relief for the family to have their loved one back with them, and to know he was safe from the destruction of war. Everyone would sleep better tonight.

• • • • • •

On the morning of February 24, 1972, Darrell Bright brought his wife, Edna, to Etta's house to give birth to their first child. Etta showed Edna to her bed where she would be giving birth while Harrison entertained Darrell in the living room. Estalee Gilliam occupied the other bed in Etta's birthing room. She was going to give birth to twins. Estalee had been with Etta for almost a week. The two women talked to one another about the excitement of seeing their new babies and rested in their beds while Etta went about her daily chores.

That night, a few minutes past midnight, Estalee began having strong labor pains. Etta was called in. Hours passed until finally at 3:55 A.M. on February 25, 1972, Estalee gave birth to the first twin. She was a breech birth, but had no major complications. Etta just barely got the umbilical cord cut and had the baby wrapped in a warm blanket before the second baby decided it was time to see the world. This one was a boy. Estalee was thrilled—

one of each gender. John and Estalee named their 6-pound, 6-ounce daughter Sandra Kay. The boy, weighing 6 pounds, 14 ounces, was named Sanford Carroll.

Later that day, at 2:20 P.M., Edna gave birth to a baby girl weighing 7 pounds, 10 ounces. Darrell and Edna named their little treasure Linda Bright.

A reporter from the local newspaper came to write the following article about the births:

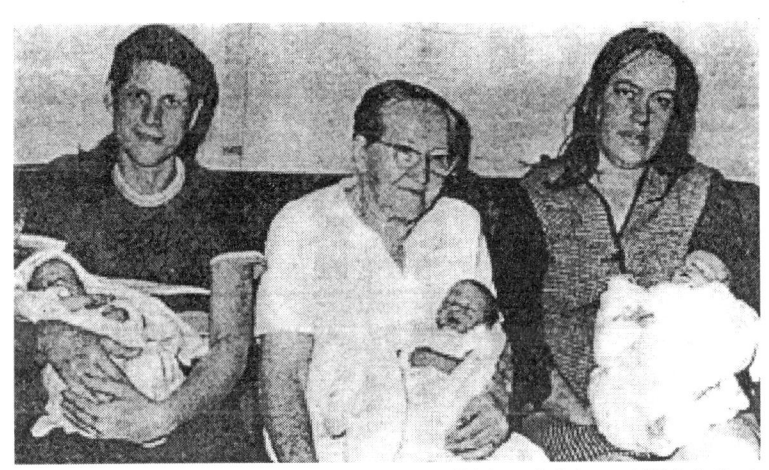

Etta "Granny" Nichols—Last of the Old-Timey Midwives

BUSY DAY—Last Friday was a busy day for Mrs. James Harrison Nichols, a midwife for over 1,000 Cocke County babies during the past 40 years. Mrs. Nichols helped deliver three babies, including a set of twins. Shown are the babies and mothers, all doing fine. From left are Mrs. Estalee Gilliam, who gave birth to twin boy and girl at 3:55 A.M. and 4 A.M.; Mrs. Nichols, holding the second of Mrs. Gilliam's twins; and Mrs. Edna Bright, the mother of a new baby girl, born at 2:20 P.M. Friday.

Fourteenth Set Of Twins Is Landmark For Local Midwife

Mrs. James Harrison Nichols reached what many people would call a landmark early Friday morning—she delivered her 14th set of twin babies and she isn't even a doctor.

The twins were born to Mrs. Estalee Gilliam, wife of Johnny C. Gilliam, Star Route, Newport, the first at 3:55 A.M. and the second one five minutes later. One was a girl weighing 6 pounds 6 ounces; and the other was a boy, tipping the scales at 6 pounds, 14 ounces.

Mrs. Nichols wasn't quite through after delivering the twins. At 2:20 P.M. on the same day she helped Mrs. Edna Bright, of Sevierville, with a baby girl weighing 7 pounds, 10 ounces.

No One Worried

But no one was worried because Mrs. Nichols doesn't hold an MD degree. Since becoming a midwife over 41 years ago, Mrs. Nichols has helped deliver over 1,026 children. The reason we say "over 1,026" is because she hasn't been counting since June, 1970.

Mrs. Nichols, the wife of James Harrison Nichols, Laurel Branch Rd., was raised with the medical profession all around her. Both her grandfather, John B. Grisby, and her father, J.L. Grisby were practicing physicians. Her grandfather practiced for about 50 years, and her father for about 30 years.

She learned from accompanying her father on house calls.

The latest babies were born in Mrs. Nichol's home where she has been practicing during the past five years. She has prepared a special room where the mother can stay until she feels ready to return home. The first baby delivered at her home was on July 17, 1967.

Whiff of Ether

Her patients are not given anesthetic. Birth is by natural childbirth and an occasional whiff of ether.

The Gilliam twins are named Sandra Kay and Sanford Carroll. Grandparents are Mr. and Mrs. Charlie Gilliam, Rt. 3, Newport; and Mr. and Mrs. Jesse Bail, Rt. 2, Cosby.

The new daughter of Mr. and Mrs. Darrell Bright is named Linda. Grandparents are Mr. and Mrs. Bruce Smith, Sevierville; and Mrs. Etta Blue of Montague, Texas.

News article and photos courtesy of The Newport Plain Talk.

On September 29, 1973, Charlotte Reese was driven to Etta's house by her husband, Hobart, to give birth to their sixth child. Etta had delivered all of the Reeses' previous children, and had delivered Charlotte also. Charlotte's first child, Shirley Jean, was born February 25, 1962; Tammy Melinda, whose middle name was named by Etta, was born October 27, 1964; Lisa Kay was an eager arrival who would not wait until her mother could get out of the car. Etta had to perform the delivery in her driveway on June 2, 1966. Charlotte did not even get her clothes off when Michael Dale was born on August 20, 1969. The fifth child, Angela Marie, was born August 7, 1971. She was named after Marie Smith Ellison.

During Charlotte's stay at Etta's for Angela's birth, another woman came to give birth in the other bed. Etta brought the woman a drink of water. For some unknown reason, the woman squirted the water through her mouth and it went all over Etta's face. This upset Etta. She stood silent and still for a moment as the water dripped from her chin, then she turned to the woman and said in an angry tone, "I've been baptized before, but I've never been sprinkled!" Etta walked over to the sink and washed her face, then left the room.

At noon on September 29, 1973, Charlotte gave birth to her sixth child. He was named James Todd.

In the Fall of 1975, Kathy Smith went to Etta's house to get a shot for strep throat. Etta was 78 years old now, and her hands shook slightly. To the person receiving one of her shots, her shaking seemed even more severe as she approached them with the needle. As Kathy stood waiting in the kitchen, she must have had a frightened look on her face because Etta grinned and said, "You ain't gonna pass out on me, are you? One of Jack Barrett's boys was here last week to get a shot, and he passed out cold as a cucumber right here on the kitchen floor before I could get the needle in, and I'd say he's about 20 years old. I had to get 'im aroused, and make 'im lean over the bed in the living room in case he did it again." Etta stood laughing as she recalled the incident.

Kathy laughed, and answered, "No, I don't think I'll pass out. I just feel weak from being sick."

"Well, let's go in here at the bed, just in case. You look pretty pale," Etta said.

Kathy made it through the ordeal okay without passing out. Etta charged Kathy $2, and told her to go home and go to bed. Although most people dreaded taking a shot from Etta, her small fee made it more bearable.

On October 14, 1976, Harrison celebrated his 80th birthday. The following day, October 15, Harrison and Etta celebrated their 60th wedding anniversary. The following Sunday, October 17, Harrison and Etta's family and friends gathered at Etta's house to honor this special occasion. Later that day a reporter from The Newport Plain Talk arrived to interview the couple. The following article appeared in the Monday addition of the paper.

Sharon Smith-Ledford

Mr., Mrs. Harrison Nichols Married Sixty Years

On Sunday, October 15, 1916, Miss Etta Grigsby, daughter of Mr. and Mrs. J. L. Grigsby became the bride of Harrison Nichols in a ceremony officiated by Squire Jimmy Jones at the home of Ishom Stinson in Del Rio.

The dreams for the future were many on that day in 1916, but not in their wildest dreams did they have visions of celebrating their 60th Wedding Anniversary, surrounded by their children, grandchildren and great-grandchildren.

On Sunday, October 17th the couple was honored with an open house at their home in Del Rio, where all their 60 married years have been spent, in observance of their 60th wedding anniversary.

To their union was born four children, Mrs. June Gilliland of Morristown; Jack Nichols, Del Rio; Belle Smith, Del Rio and Emily Jones, deceased. They are blessed with 13 living grandchildren and 16 living great-grandchildren.

Mr. Nichols, who celebrated his 80th birthday on October 14th is a retired farmer.

Mrs. Nichols has contributed to the health care of young mothers in Cocke County and surrounding counties for 47 years as a practicing Mid-wife.

In her little clinic, white and immaculate at the rear of her home, she has delivered approximately 1,500 babies, "I stopped counting in 1970," she said, and has never lost one." Only three of that number were born dead," the mid-wife said.

"No, I will never retire, but of course that's up to the Lord, as long as he gives me strength and good health I'll be delivering babies," Mrs. Nichols said with that ever present smile on her face.

During those 47 years, Mr. Nichols has been present entertaining expecting fathers, waiting for that first cry. "He has always gone along with me in my work for he knew I was never one to sit around and twiddle my thumbs," she said.

On Sunday, Mrs. Nichols was lovely in a beige and aqua street length dress complimented by a corsage of bronze and yellow mums as she and her husband greeted their guests.

The serving table was covered with a white linen cloth and centered with a large anniversary cake decorated with clusters of orange sugar flowers. Punch was served from a crystal bowl. Nuts and party mints were also served to the many guests who called between the appointed hours of 2-5 P.M.

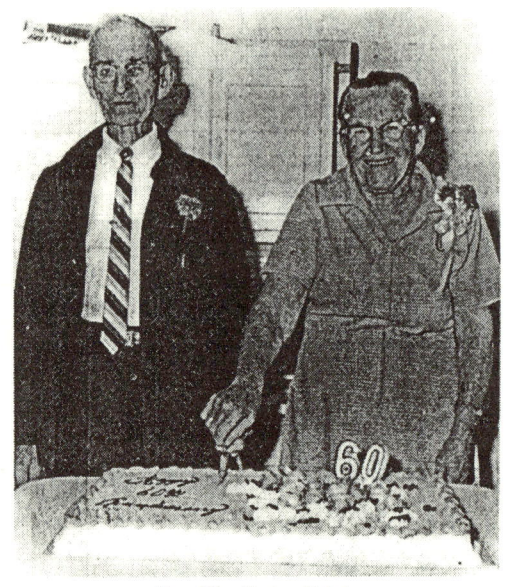

Mr. and Mrs. Harrison Nichols

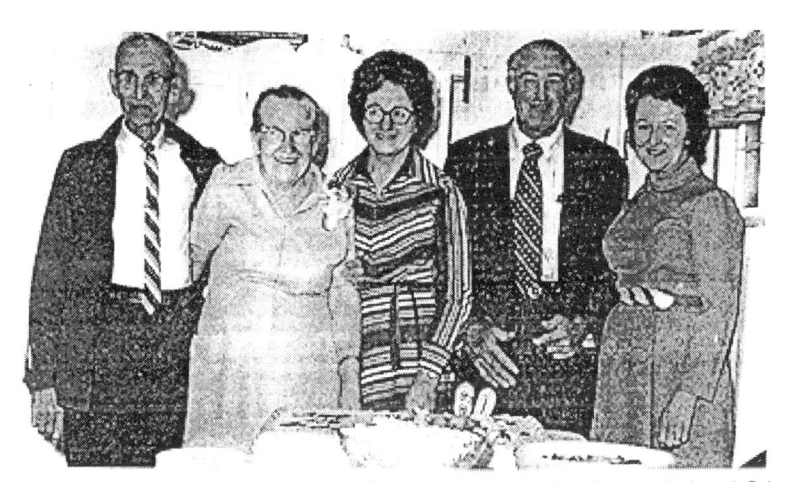

Etta "Granny" Nichols—Last of the Old-Timey Midwives

MR. AND MRS. HARRISON NICHOLS with their children at the Open House held on Sunday at ther home in Del Rio, in observance of their 00th wedding anniversary. From left are Mr. and Mrs. Nichols, June Gilliland, Jack Nichols and Belle Smith. **(Photo by Elliott.)**

News article and photos courtesy of The Newport Plain Talk.

Etta continued delivering babies throughout the following years, one of which was born to Eugene Pack, whom Etta also had delivered, and his wife, Betty, from Bat Harbor. Their son, Terry Eugene, was born November 10, 1976. He weighed 5 pounds and 1 ounce. This was a difficult birth for Betty because it was a dry birth. Etta had also delivered their oldest daughter, Lena Michelle, born on September 6, 1973. She weighed 5 pounds.

Etta's granddaughter, Lynda, was already three weeks late from the due date the doctor had given her as the date she would deliver her fourth child. Lynda had decided to let Etta deliver this one. The other three, Renina, Darren, and Lisa had all been born in the hospital. Lynda and her husband, Edd Burgin, owned a house on Dry Fork, about three miles away from Etta. On June 26, 1978, Lynda went to have a check-up at Etta's house. After examining her, Etta told her it would not be long. That night Lynda had her first pain around 11:30. Lynda called her mother, "Mom, I'll be by shortly to drop off the kids. I just had my first pain."

"Oh, really?! Well, I'll be waiting. Bring 'em on." Belle answered.

Lynda woke her husband and told him it was time. Edd reacted as the "normal frantic father" in this type of situation. While Lynda was in the bathroom taking her hair down, Edd woke up the children and got them in the car. Lynda's pains were coming stronger and closer now. After leaving the kids with their grandmother, Edd drove Lynda to Etta's. It was now 1:15 A.M. Emily's daughter, Debbie, was there staying with Etta to have her first baby. What a thrill for Etta to have the opportunity to deliver two of her great-grandchildren so close together. Debbie was asleep in the other bedroom when Lynda arrived and never woke up when Lynda came in. Etta and Edd helped Lynda to the birthing room in the back of the house. Edd stayed in the room with Lynda and held her hand during the delivery.

"I told you it wouldn't be long," Etta chuckled. "You're doin' so good. Just bare down all you can when you get a pain," Etta continued.

At 2:30 A.M. on June 27, 1978, a little baby girl made her entrance into the world. Etta took her newborn great-granddaughter into her arms ever so gently, and wiped her clean as she talked sweet baby talk to the new arrival. After weighing her, she placed her in Lynda's arms. Lynda's heart immediately filled with love for her new daughter, the kind of love that only a mother and her child can know. Edd had never experienced anything quite like this before. He was in awe of everything he had just witnessed. The proud parents named their 8-pound, 15-ounce daughter, Sheri Melaine Burgin.

The next morning Debbie got out of bed and was astonished to find Lynda had given birth there that night. "But, I never heard a thing!" Debbie said surprisingly. "Didn't you scream any, or let out a holler, or anything?"

"No. I got along better here than I did at the hospital when I had my others," Lynda answered. "Mamaw was so sweet, and she just coaxed me right through the whole thing. I can't even tell I've had a baby this morning," Lynda giggled.

"Boy, I hope I get along as well as you did," Debbie said.

Lynda stayed with Etta that day, then went home the following morning to introduce the newest member of the Burgin family to her siblings.

Five days after Lynda gave birth, Debbie went into labor during the afternoon of July 2, 1978. She had been having false labor pains every day since Lynda had left.

Etta told Debbie, "This is going to be a dry birth. If you had gone to the hospital they would probably do a cesarean. I'll save you from having a big scar."

"Well, I appreciate that," Debbie answered.

Etta knew her granddaughter was scared to death. This was her first child, and she would have a lot of extra pain because of it being a dry birth. Etta began telling stories about other women who had come to her, trying to take Debbie's mind off her pain. "There was this one woman who came here to have a baby, and I went in the other room to get something, and when I came back she was gone. Then I heard her screamin' outside. I run to the door and there she was, runnin' along the creek bed waving her arms all over the place and screaming to wake the dead! I hollered at Harrison and he run out back and got a limb off a tree and went down there and told her if she didn't get back to the house he was goin' to use that hickory on her. She finally came back. I asked her why she did that, and she said she was runnin' to try to get away from the pain."

Debbie laughed as Etta continued, "And then there was this other woman who come to me thinkin' she was only going to have one baby, and I thought so, too, 'cause I could only hear one heart beat. Anyway, after she had the baby she kept havin' pains. We both thought it was just the afterbirth trying to come out, and then, all of a sudden, another baby just shot out of there. I was standing at the end of the bed, and I caught it. Boy, was she surprised!" Etta laughed.

Etta continued telling stories until Debbie was in the last stages of delivery.

"Oh, it hurts, Mamaw. Am I going to die?" Debbie asked.

Etta laughed. "No, honey, you're not gonna die. Every woman who gives birth thinks she's gonna die, but they all get through it," Etta answered. Etta placed a pillow under Debbie's back to help relieve the back cramps she was having, then continued talking to her while Debbie's friend, Karen Sayne, held a cotton ball of ether under Debbie's nose.

"Give me that bottle of ether and let me drink it!" Debbie said only half joking.

Etta felt the head of the baby with her fingers. "He's havin' a hard time gettin' out of there. His head is goin' toward the rectum instead of where it should be goin'," Etta said. Etta used her fingers to pull the baby's head up where it should be, then at 11:40 P.M. Debbie gave birth to an 8-pound baby boy. She named him Joshua Shane.

Debbie stayed with her grandmother for several days after the birth before going back home where she lived in Morristown. Etta would miss having Debbie and the baby there.

• • • • • •

In March of 1978 Etta received a book in the mail entitled <u>Redneck Mothers, Good Ol' Girls and Other Southern Belles</u>, written by Sharon McKern. Mrs. McKern had interviewed Etta sometime earlier to include Etta's story in her book. Etta's story of how she became a midwife appeared on pages 195-200 in the book.

Etta's children and grandchildren were thrilled with all the recognition she was receiving about her life's work, but Etta paid no attention to her growing popularity. She just considered herself to be a down-to-earth country woman who did all she could to help others.

On May 1, 1979, Donald Jenkins drove his wife, Pauline, from White Pine, Tennessee, to Etta's to give birth. "We heard about you through a friend of ours, Ann Rhines," Donald told Etta. "She said you are real good at delivering babies."

"Well, I do all the good Lord will let me do. I try to do a good job," Etta answered.

Etta led Pauline to the birthing room while Donald waited anxiously in the living room with Harrison. Thirty minutes later, around 7 P.M. the sound of a baby's cry filled the air. Pauline gave birth to a 7-pound baby boy. They named him Christopher Michael.

Pauline was having trouble getting the afterbirth out, and after examining her, Etta thought it best to take Pauline to the hospital, in case surgery was necessary. Pauline left her new born son with Etta while she was in the hospital. One and a half days later Donald and Pauline returned for their son. Etta would not accept more than $10 for payment. She told them she only did half the job and would not feel good charging them the entire $15. Donald paid Etta then took his family home.

Father's Day, June 17, 1979, Debbie Owens Stokley started having labor pains with her second child early Sunday morning. She went into the bedroom to tell her husband, Tony, to get up and get ready to take her to the hospital. Tony thought he had plenty of time, since the birth of their first child, Brandy, took so long. He got out of bed and went to the bathroom to shave. Meanwhile, Debbie's pains were getting closer and harder. Debbie kept calling to her husband to hurry up. Finally, Tony was ready. Tony and Debbie were going to leave Brandy with Tony's mother, Polly Shelton, who lived on Blue Mill Road, on their way to the hospital. When they arrived at Polly's house they all went inside. Suddenly, without warning, Debbie's water broke. Debbie started to panic. Polly told her to go in the bedroom and lie down so she could check her. Debbie did as Polly asked. Polly went out into the hallway after checking Debbie and yelled to her daughter, Sherry, to bring some plastic and blankets...the baby was coming now.

"What am I going to do?!" Tony asked frantically.

"Go get Mrs. Nichols!" Polly screamed.

Tony ran hysterically outside and jumped in the car. The tires screeched loudly as Tony took off up the road. In Tony's frantic state of mind, he did not realize until he was halfway to Etta's that the car he jumped in was not his. It belonged to a friend of Polly's who was there visiting. Tony continued up the dirt road leading to Etta's house. Normally, Etta would have been gone to church with Harrison at this time, but it turned out Etta was home waiting on a patient who had come to her from Dandridge to give birth. Tony's car went sideways as he entered Etta's driveway. Once stopped, Tony jumped from the car and ran up the front steps.

"Mrs. Nichols, you've got to come with me. My wife is giving birth right now! We need your help!"

Etta grabbed her medical bag and hurried to the car with Tony. Tony's driving was somewhat reckless as he maneuvered the car around the curves. Fresh gravel had just been poured on the road a few days earlier, making the handling of the car even more difficult. Tony was taking the curves sideways as he rushed to get Etta to his wife in time. He looked over at Etta and asked, "Am I scaring you?"

"Keep it between the ditches, and lay it to it!" Etta answered.

Upon arriving at Polly's, Etta went to the bedroom where Debbie was. Debbie was in a full panic now, knowing she was going to go through natural childbirth. Etta knew she had to get Debbie's emotions under control before she could help her. Etta spoke in a stern voice to Debbie, "Turn around in this bed, and act like you're going to have a baby!"

Debbie did as Etta ordered her to do. Polly had called the Rescue Squad from Newport to come up, in case Tony did not find Etta at home. They arrived 15 minutes or so after Etta got there. The members of the Rescue Squad just stood back in the corner of the bedroom and watched as Etta worked with Debbie.

Debbie had been pushing for close to an hour now. Polly stood by Debbie holding her hand and kissing her forehead. Tony had drunk 26 cups of coffee during the hour, between the times he was not putting cold cloths on Debbie's head, or putting chapstick on her lips.

Tony's pacing back and forth through the hallway apparently started to get on Etta's nerves. She looked up at Tony and said in a firm voice, "If you want to help her, then get up on this bed and let her pull to you when she has a pain."

Tony did as Etta instructed.

"Come on, Deb! You can do it! If you can live with Tony, you can do anything!" Polly said. Polly suggested using the rescuer's backboard to put under Debbie to help support her better during her contractions. Etta agreed that would help. Once Debbie had the backboard in place, she gave a good strong push, and at 11:25 A.M. the baby was born. Silence fell over the room as they noticed the baby had the umbilical cord around its neck and was turning blue. Etta hurried to remove the cord as family members stood around her holding their breath. Etta removed the cord successfully and the baby started crying.

Tony leaned over to take a look at his newborn son. "I want you to look at the manhood on that boy!" Tony said proudly.

Etta burst into laughter over Tony's straightforward statement, and soon laughter filled the room as everyone let out a sigh of relief. Debbie had given birth to an 8-pound baby boy. She and Tony named their son Trinity Royal Stokley. Tony paid Etta her regular fee of $15, then drove Etta home.

The next day Debbie called her best friend, Sharon Kay. "Guess what. Your grandmother delivered my baby yesterday."

"She did?! But I thought you were going to have it in the hospital," Sharon answered.

"Well, I would have, but Tony thought he had to shave before taking me. When I got to Polly's my water broke and we had to get Mrs. Nichols to come down."

"Well, what about that! My grandmother delivered my best friend's baby. That just thrills me to death," Sharon told her.

Debbie told Sharon every detail of her experience. "I was afraid, but Mrs. Nichols knew what to do and how to do it. We're both just fine, thanks to her."

A little over one month later Etta's granddaughter, Sandra, went into labor at her home in Morristown. She immediately called her sister, Debbie, to drive her to Etta's to have the baby.

Debbie arrived at Sandra's house in about 15 minutes. The rain was pouring down so hard Debbie could barely see the road, which forced her to drive very slowly. Debbie was scared Sandra would have the baby before they reached Del Rio. She kept telling Sandra all the way up the road, "I don't know nothin' about birthin' no babies. You wait 'til we get there."

When Debbie and Sandra reached Del Rio the creeks were coming out of their banks into the road. Debbie proceeded on with caution through the water. The two made it safely to their grandmother's house about 5 P.M. Saturday evening and hurried inside. Sandra kept having contractions for several more hours. Debbie stayed in the room with her sister to offer any help she could give. At 10 P.M. on Saturday night, July 21, 1979, Sandra gave birth to a 10-pound, 2-ounce baby boy with no complications. Sandra named her new son Larry Dustin Brooks. This was Etta's sixth great-grandchild that she had been fortunate enough to help bring into the world. The next day Sandra's husband, dad, and her other child, Brett Wayne, came to Etta's to see her and the baby. Sandra was feeling so good she decided to go back with them, but not before sitting down and eating dinner with her grandmother. Sandra was not going to miss Etta's good cooking. After dinner the happy family returned to Morristown with their newest little member.

During the second week of March, 1981, Carson Brewer, a reporter from The Knoxville News-Sentinel newspaper came to interview Etta. On Sunday, March 15, 1981, the following article appeared in the Sunday addition of that paper.

Sharon Smith-Ledford

Slabtown Midwife Has Delivered

Carson Brewer

ALTHOUGH INFLATION has rocketed the cost of medical care and nearly everything else in the past decade, the fee for delivering a baby in Slabtown remains the same as it's been for 40 years—$15.

You never heard of Slabtown? Of course you have. The late opera star Grace Moore was born there in 1901—when the fee probably was much less than $15.

Slabtown is in South Cocke County, south of the French Broad River, south of Del Rio. It is on Big Creek and its small hurrying tributaries. Chickens, turkeys, guinea fowl, domestic ducks and even a few half-wild Mallards forage along the creeks and narrow roads. The most obvious piece of landscape in the area is Max Patch Mountain.

Though the Slabtown area is within the general boundaries of Cherokee National Forest, several families live there on private inholdings.

One of those pieces of private land is the tract of 35 to 40 acres on Laurel Branch owned by Harrison and Etta Nichols, 84 and 83 years old, respectively. Etta Nichols is a midwife, has been for 51 years.

When I was writing about midwifery in December, I asked some of the nurses in the state Health Department whether there was an old-time "granny woman" left in East Tennessee. That's when Lynne Smith-Newport, the state's family planning nurse practitioner for East Tennessee, told me about Etta Nichols. Most of her mountain neighbors call her "Etter." Nothing's wrong with that. The elite of Boston speak similarly. Remember how President John Kennedy said "Cuber" for Cuba?

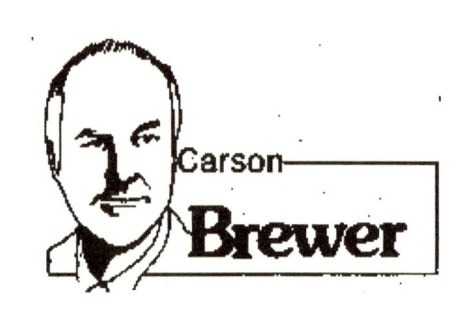

Lynne took me to see Etta Nichols one recent chilly morning. The top of Max Patch was white with hoarfrost. A fire burned in the Nichols fireplace.

The green walls of the Nichols' living room are half-covered with pictures of children. Many are of her own grandchildren, great-grandchildren and perhaps even of her two great-great-grandchildren. Many others are pictures of children Mrs. Nichols helped bring into the world.

How many has she delivered?

She didn't know exactly. But when she counted about a year, ago, the number was nearly 2000. So she thinks it's more than 2000 now. She said she delivered more last year than in any previous year. She delivered four during one recent week.

Why has her business picked up? Because there are fewer midwives and "doctors won't go out," she said. She didn't mention another likely factor: Her $15 fee is only a fraction of the cost of having a baby in a hospital under care of an obstetrician.

In all those 2000-plus births, Mrs. Nichols said, she's never lost a mother. She's lost about 10 babies. Six of these were three sets of premature twins. Another was a stillborn twin; the other twin lived.

She has, satisfied customers. One mother has come to her for nine deliveries. One woman who kept coming back year after year got some simple family-planning advice: "Tell him to sleep on the roof," Lynne quoted Mrs. Nichols as telling the woman. Mrs. Nichols seemed embarrassed to discuss such matters with a strange man.

Though her fee is $15, one happy father recently pressed $200 on her. She said it was because she delivered the baby on her and Harrison's 64th wedding anniversary, Oct. 15. She gave part of the big fee to a woman who helped her. She needed help because she'd suffered a slight injury in working with one of her milk goats.

When she was a child, she wanted to be a nurse, "but I never got to go to school." So she decided to be a midwife. Her grandfather, John B. Grigsby, was a physician, a man with a proper medical degree. Her father, John L Grigsby, had no medical degree. But he learned from his father and doctored anyway. She went on calls with him and learned from him. "He told me a lot I never forgot."

She says the secret of being a good midwife is patience. Lynne Smith agrees. Lynne says

Etta "Granny" Nichols—Last of the Old-Timey Midwives

women like to have Mrs. Nichols deliver their babies because she doesn't rush them.

Mrs. Nichols looks patient. She's not too large and not too small. Her country woman's voice is calm and gentle. She gently massages a woman in labor, helps the tissues to stretch without tearing, does no cutting to widen the opening.

For years, she went to the homes of expectant mothers. Sometimes she walked eight or 10 miles, often in snow over her shoetops. Sometimes she rode a horse.

But in about 1967 or 1968, circumstances changed. Both Mrs. Nichols' mother and her husband's mother became ill and had to come and live in the Nichols home. Mrs. Nichols had to stop going on baby calls. The expectant mothers started coming to her.

I was puzzled. Where in this small house would a woman have a baby? The house has four rooms. There is the living room, which also is Mrs. Nichols' bedroom. She likes to sleep there to be near the phone. Harrison sleeps in another bedroom. Then there is the combination kitchen-dining room.

The fourth room is the birthing room. It has two narrow beds. Next to the wall between them is an incubator. Lynne said the Health Department gave it to Mrs. Nichols 11 or 12 years ago. Lynne told Mrs. Nichols then that she should place premature babies smaller than 5.5 pounds in the incubator and then phone the Health Department in Newport.

With the help of doctors at the Valentine-Shults Hospital & Clinic in Newport, Lynne would arrange for the premature baby to be admitted to University Hospital's Intensive Care Nursery. And the Cocke County Rescue Squad would take mother and baby there. The smallest baby Mrs. Nichols ever delivered weighed 2.5 pounds and it's still living.

Mrs. Nichols got her baby scales with green stamps. She bakes the sheets used in the room in her range oven or irons them with a hot iron. This to kill germs, Lynne explains. She puts silver nitrate drops in the infants' eyes to prevent infection.

Some mothers almost don't make it to the Nichols house. Mrs. Nichols delivered one infant in the car in the yard. And one recent Sunday night she and Harrison were at the Bridgeport Freewill Baptist Church when a young Morristown man rushed into the church to get her. His wife was outside in the car, about to have a baby any minute.

Mrs. Nichols quickly got the house key from Harrison and went home in the car with the husband and expectant mama. They got her onto one of the beds. The husband yanked off one of her shoes and Mrs. Nichols pulled off the other. The baby arrived the instant the shoes were off. Mrs. Nichols said she'd have had the baby earlier if she hadn't had the "slow misery."

What's that? It's prolonged labor caused by the cord being wrapped around the baby's neck. This one was wrapped twice around the neck.

Though Etta Nichols has lost no mothers, and few babies, it seems reasonable to believe that birth in a modern hospital would be safer for the babies. But Mrs. Nichols very likely operates the best $15 baby delivery service in Tennessee. And this is a compelling reason why hundreds of expectant mothers from as far away as Knox, Jefferson, Sevier and Greene Counties go to her.

And if somebody doesn't have $15, that's all right, too. There was the woman from up East who married a Tennessee mountain man and came here to live with him. She got pregnant. She and her husband separated. Her husband's parents brought her to the Nichols home three weeks before the baby came. She stayed on six weeks after it came. She ate at the Nichols table. She bummed chewing tobacco from Harrison. When she left, Harrison told her she owed a $40 board bill and $5 for tobacco. She laughed as if she thought he was joking.

"We never got a brownie," Mrs. Nichols said.

She told the story with mixed mirth and irony. No bitterness.

Would she take the woman back if she came back pregnant again?

"I'd take care of her again. I've never asked one yet if she had the money. I've never turned one away."

News articles and photos courtesy of The Knoxville News-Sentinel.

Sharon Smith-Ledford

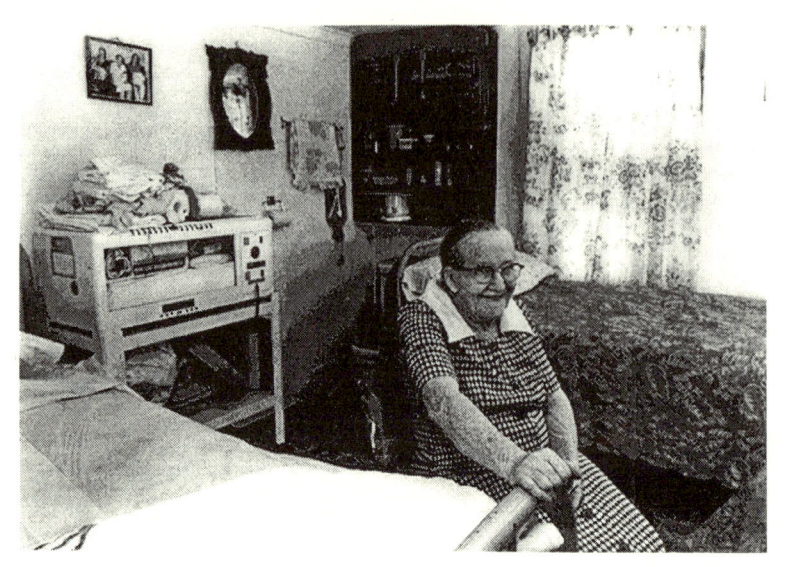

Etta sits in her delivery room to pose for The Knoxville News Sentinel.

On July 4, 1981, Etta lost her youngest brother, J. L., to cancer. He was survived by his wife, Loiree, his son, Michael, his daughter, Dianne, and four grandchildren. J. L. was buried in the Clark Cemetery on Midway Road.

Thursday night, August 20, 1981, Lawrence Green called Etta to tell her he was on his way to bring his wife, Linda, to give birth to twins. Etta had delivered the Greens' first child, Jessica Loyetta, the previous year on April 27, so the Greens felt comfortable allowing Etta to deliver their twins. As always, Etta told funny stories to her patients to try to keep their mind off their pain. After Linda arrived and was settled in the birthing room, Etta started in on her story-telling.

"There was this black married couple, and the wife was cheating on the husband. Well, she got pregnant by a white man. The woman didn't know how she was going to explain the color of the baby to her husband, so one hot summer day in mid-July the woman told her husband she was craving snow. He told her he couldn't get her any snow in July. She looked at her husband very disappointedly and told him, 'Well, don't blame me if this baby turns out to be white.'"

Linda laughed for the longest time at the story Etta told her. Around 9:30 P.M. Linda started having hard pains. At 12:20 A.M. on the 21st of August, the first twin was born. It was a boy weighing 4 pounds and 8 ounces. Linda had a hard time giving birth to the baby because he was a breech birth, and a dry birth. Ninety minutes later Linda gave birth to the second twin. This one was a girl, weighing 4 pounds and 5 ounces. The twins were named Justin Lawrence, and Jennifer Lynn Green.

Etta took the twins to bed with her. She told Linda she wanted to make sure they stayed warm, and Linda needed to sleep to regain her strength.

The Newport Plain Talk newspaper had told Etta they wanted to do a story the next time she delivered twins, so later that day Etta called them with the news of the twins' birth. Jeff Wallace was sent to Etta's to do the interview. The following article appeared in the next addition of the paper:

Del Rio Midwife Keeps Delivering The Babies

By Jeff Wallace

The average woman, when planning how and where she is going to give birth, thinks of a hospital waiting at the end of a smooth state highway with doctors and nurses who are ready to attend to her.

There are only a few mothers-to-be that would drive down a dirt road at midnight to find someone living in a house miles from any main highway to deliver their baby.

But that is exactly how one Cocke County woman decided she wanted her child to be born.

After Linda Green went into labor late Thursday night, her husband Larry drove her into a rural area near Del Rio where Etta Nichols, who had been called and told that "it is time" by the Greens, was prepared to deliver the baby. At 12:20 A.M., Mrs. Green gave birth to a baby boy. At 1:50 A.M., Mrs. Green gave birth to a baby girl. Both of the twins were delivered with the aid of the lady best known in east Cocke County as "the midwife Nichols."

Being 84 years old has neither stopped nor slowed down Mrs. Nichols from delivering babies. For more than 52 years she has been a midwife, helping bring babies into the world at all hours of the night and day.

"A while back somebody asked me when I am going to retire," Mrs. Nichols said. "I told them I'm not going to quit until I'm dead flat on my back and my toes are sticking straight up in the air."

Mrs. Nichols said couples from as far away as Cleveland, Tenn. and Marshall, N.C. search her out when the time comes for their babies to be born. She said she used to make house calls, "but now they just come to me."

In 52 years of being a midwife, Mrs. Nichols has delivered more than 2,000 babies, and the twins born to the Greens Friday were not the first set delivered by the midwife.

"Oh, I've delivered many twins," she explained. "It's been in the teens of times. But I've never delivered any triplets. I hope that sometime I get to deliver a set of triplets."

Mrs. Nichols explained that more than anything else, a midwife must exercise patience. She said when she was younger several women asked her to train them to be a midwife. She added that most of the women did not have the time, stamina or patience needed to be a midwife and gave up soon after she started telling them about what it entails. "These days," Mrs. Nichols said, nobody asks about being a midwife.

"In all my days, I've never lost a mother," she said. "Now, there have been occasions when I nearly lost the father. I remember one that fainted plumb out on the floor."

Some of the most sad occasions Mrs. Nichols recalls have been when babies she has delivered are stillborn.

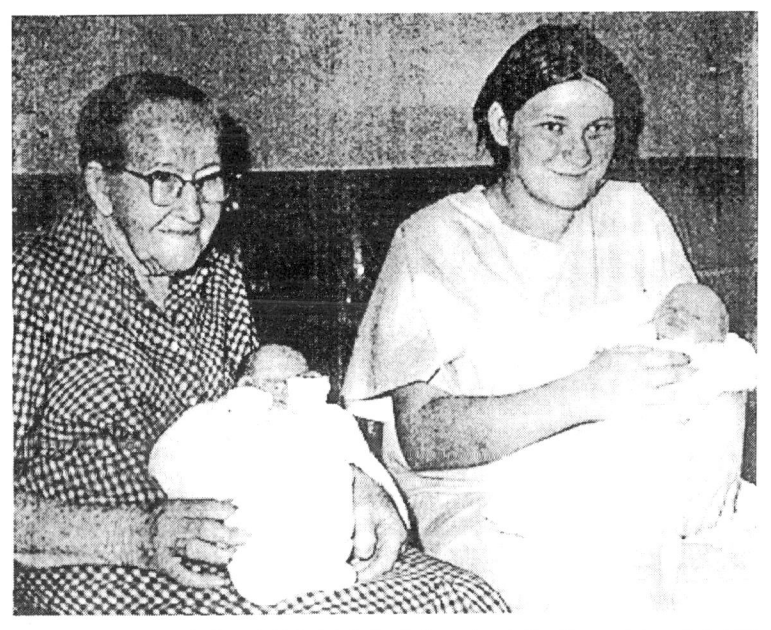

Etta "Granny" Nichols—Last of the Old-Timey Midwives

Etta Nichols, left, with Linda Green hold the twin babies that were born to Mrs. Green only hours before this photograph was taken. Mrs. Nichols says she delivered more than 2,000 babies in the 52 years she has been a midwife. This is not the first set of twins she has delivered. Mrs. Nichols says when "it is time," some parents-to-be will call her while others simply show up on her door step. **(photo by Jeff Wallace)**

"I've lost a few that were born premature," she said. "Those I sent down to UT (University of Tennessee) Hospital in Knoxville hoping they could do something for them. I've delivered a few that just drawed a breath or two before dying."

Mrs. Nichols said she had planned to be a nurse when she was young. As a teenager, she followed her father, who was a doctor, around as he made his calls. She said he delivered many babies and added that it was from him that she learned to deliver babies herself. Unfortunately, she never became a certified nurse, but that did not stop her from delivering babies." I delivered a baby right in the middle of town one time in Newport," Mrs. Nichols explained.

"I don't think it could ever get on my nerves. Some people don't believe that. I'd be just as happy if I delivered one every day and every night," she said.

Mrs. Nichols has never delivered more than three babies in one 24-hour period. The day she delivered three, she assisted in the birth of a set of twins earlier in the day and later delivered another baby.

"There have been plenty of days that I've delivered two babies, though," she said.

Mrs. Nichols said she first realized how long she has been a midwife when she delivered a baby boy, and later found out that it was the grandson of a woman she had delivered almost 50 years earlier.

"Some of them will call ahead of time and others will just show up on my doorstep," Mrs. Nichols explained. "I just do my best to help the mother give birth to her beautiful baby."

News article and photos courtesy of The Newport Plain Talk.

Etta got a special present on her 85th birthday on May 19, 1982. She delivered a little Mexican baby boy, Ricardo Lopez, weighing 7 pounds and 12 ounces. Ricardo was the third Mexican baby she had delivered. The following article appeared in <u>The Newport Plain Talk</u> telling about the happy occasion:

Etta "Granny" Nichols—Last of the Old-Timey Midwives

Shares Joy On Birthday

By Shirley Elliott

Mrs. Harrison Nichols, Del Rio midwife, delivered her first baby 52 years ago. At age 85 she is still on the job and loving every minute of it. Wednesday, May 19 at 10:25 A.M. on her 85th birthday she delivered Ricardo Lopez, son of Mr. and Mrs. Joaquin Lopez of Route 1, Bybee. Ricardo and his parents are Mexican.

"I wanted to be a nurse, but I never did get to go to school so I did the next best thing—I became a midwife," Mrs. Nichols said with a glow in her eye.

She said her father, John L. Grigsby and her grandfather, John B. Grigsby, were doctors and on two or three occasions she went with her father on house calls. "I loved the work and that is when I knew I wanted to be a nurse," she said.

She remembers the day she began her career as a midwife as if it were yesterday. "My first baby was still nursing I remember; so it has to be 52 years ago. Word came that Editha Morrow was in labor. As soon as Harrison (her husband) got home I headed up the road and later delivered her baby," she said. That baby grew up to be Bud Morrow.

How many babies have you delivered in those 52 years? "I can't be for sure, but it will be well over 2,000. I haven't counted them up in two years, I just haven't had the time. I keep records, you know, and when I get time I'll count and know for sure."

She related that little Ricardo, who weighed seven pounds and twelve ounces at birth, was the third Mexican baby she has delivered. Where did you get training to be a mid-

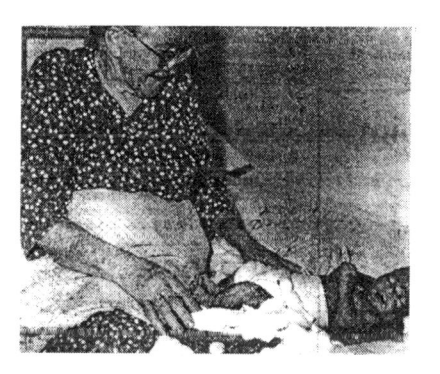

Mrs. Harrison Nichols, Del Rio midwife, smiles her special smile at Ricardo Lopez, whom she delivered on her 85th birthday Wednesday, following his bath on Thursday morning. Mrs. Nichols has delivered over 2,000 babies in her career as a midwife which spans 52 years. **(photo by Shirley Elliott)**

wife? "I picked up some things from my father and I have read some, but mostly I just did it. I hadn't read anything about it when I delivered my first baby."

The smallest baby she ever delivered weighed one and one half pounds. "And you know, that baby lived," she said with a smile. The largest baby she has delivered was a 14 pounder. "I have delivered some weighing 11 pounds, but generally they weigh between seven and nine pounds.

She said she had had several women come to her, wanting to learn how to be a midwife. "I tell them that in order to be a good midwife you have to have patience and you have to keep your courage. You know I don't give shots or anything and sometimes labor is long and it gets rough, so I tell them that patience is the key to being a good midwife."

"Some mothers go back home in a few hours after the baby is born, but they are welcome to stay as long as they want to, usually it is two or three days. You know some are up smoking cigarettes an hour after the baby is born, but I make them come in here (the living room) for smoke is bad for the baby's lungs and I don't want my babies breathing it," she said.

Mrs. Nichols has a room off her kitchen that she uses only for labor and delivery. There are two beds in the room that are snow white.

Noting how well little Ricardo was sleeping as he lay in Mrs. Nichols' arms, she said, "I put him on goat's milk. The milk is real good for babies. They sleep so well and they don't spit up. His mother didn't want to nurse him so I just put him on goat's milk," she said. She went on to say she has goats and churned the milk. "It makes the best buttermilk you ever drank," the midwife said.

Mrs. Nichols said she has delivered about 15 sets of twins, but never any triplets. "I want to deliver triplets before I leave here so bad I can taste it," she said.

When will you stop delivering babies? When my toes are sticking up," was the reply.

"If you see anybody down there that are having triplets tell them to come up here and let me deliver them."

News article and photos courtesy of The Newport Plain Talk.

Etta had delivered over 2,000 babies, according to her last count. On July 29, 1983, Etta added another delivery to her count. Joyce Turner Smelcer, wife of Kelvin Smelcer, arrived at Etta's with her mother, Peggy Baxter, and her sister, Jan Baxter around 6 A.M. Hours passed, and everyone was about to sit down to eat some pinto beans and cornbread for lunch when Joyce went into hard labor. Peggy helped her daughter to the bed in the birthing room. Etta told Joyce to start pushing. Joyce was going to have a dry birth, so Etta used petroleum jelly to lubricate the birth canal. One of Joyce's pains was so intense it caused her to black out for a moment. When the next hard pain came Joyce jumped.

Etta hollered at her, "Don't do that!"

Joyce tried to remain still during the contractions that followed. At 1:25 P.M. Joyce gave birth to a baby boy, weighing 7 pounds and 8 ounces. She named him Seth Anthony Smelcer.

Joyce was planning on feeding her baby with a bottle, but Etta made her feelings of bottle feeding very clear. Etta looked at the baby and said, "Your mama better give you the tity before she loses you." Then Etta spoke to Joyce, "If you insist on bottle feeding, then the next best thing to breast milk is goat's milk."

"Well, I don't have any goats, so I guess you've convinced me to breast feed," Joyce answered.

Joyce stayed with Etta overnight then left around noon the next day. She forced Etta to accept $50 as payment. Etta did not want to accept that much money.

"You're the sweetest thing, Granny. I've really enjoyed my stay with you. Please take the money," Joyce said. Etta smiled gratefully and put the money in her apron pocket, then Joyce left with her new baby boy.

Several weeks later, on August 18, 1983, Kathy Thomas came to Etta from Newport to have her second child. Etta had delivered Kathy's first baby, Taren, the previous year on August 8. Kathy's mother, Sue Hazel Sutton, came with Kathy and held her hand during the delivery.

After several hours of hard labor, Etta said, "Push, Honey, it's comin' out."

Kathy pushed with all her strength and gave birth to a 6 pound baby boy. She named him, Travis. During Kathy's stay Etta tried to get Kathy to drink some goat's milk, but after one sip Kathy decided she did not like it. Etta found that amusing. Kathy tried to pay Etta, but she would not accept any money. After spending two days with Etta, Kathy and her baby returned to their home in Newport.

On October 10, 1983, both The Knoxville Journal, and The Newport Plain Talk did a story about Deborah Ann Hamilton, who resided in LaFollette, coming to Etta to give birth. Deborah's daughter, Pamela, had cancer. Deborah and her husband, Larry T. Hamilton, were involved in a court battle to prevent any treatments from being given to Pamela, due to their religious beliefs. The Hamilton's court case had been receiving much attention from the television media, as well as many surrounding newspapers. The following is the article which was published in The Newport Plain Talk:

Sharon Smith-Ledford

Cancer victim's mother seeks refuge in Cocke

By Shirley Elliott

The tranquillity of the mountains surrounds Mrs. Larry (Deborah) Hamilton as she awaits the arrival of her first child in Del Rio. As she talked to me Saturday morning she was busy crocheting a sweater for the baby.

Deborah and her husband, Rev. Hamilton, are involved in a bitter court battle to prevent cancer treatments for his daughter Pamela. "It sure is nice to get away from the TV cameras and reporters," she said.

The family resides in LaFollette where Rev. Hamilton is pastor of the Church of God of the Union Assembly, Inc.

It was in July that Pamela, a 7th grader, went into a Knoxville hospital to have a broken leg set. When doctors operated to put a pin in the leg, they discovered a malignant tumor. The broken leg, Deborah said, was a result of the cancer. At this time the family was told of the avenues open to them, the treatment and the effects of treatment. "My husband explained everything to Pamela all about the treatment and everything before she left the hospital and Pamela told him she didn't want the treatment—that she just wanted to go home. She was scared to death of them (treatments)," Deborah said.

She said the Department of Human Service visited their home on two occasions and "then the whole thing just blew out of proportion," she said.

They gave us 30 days to get an attorney and said they would get a court-appointed attorney. "My husband told them to forget it that we would get our own attorney. The next thing we knew we got an order telling us they were picking her up in 48 hours. You know on that short order it was hard to get an attorney because that didn't give them time to prepare the case, but we went to Knoxville and found James A. H. Bell who agreed to take the case.

"We have never signed anything for Pamela to have the cancer treatments," Deborah added.

Pamela is at present a patient at Children's Hospital, Knoxville, taking her second round of cancer treatments. "She has a tutor who started last week and she will help her keep up with her school work. We hope to take her home in the next few weeks and a nurse will come to the house to check her," she said.

The Hamiltons' appeal has been denied by the State Supreme Court. "We do have alternatives, but at this point I am not sure what our next step will be," Deborah said.

The size of Pamela's tumor, which is located on the outside of her leg near the hip area, has been called everything from the size of a football to the size of a watermelon, and Deborah said this description had also been blown out of proportion. Holding up her hands forming a circle, she said the tumor was bigger than a baseball, but certainly not as big as a football.

Rev. Hamilton has three sons ages 14, 7, and 3.

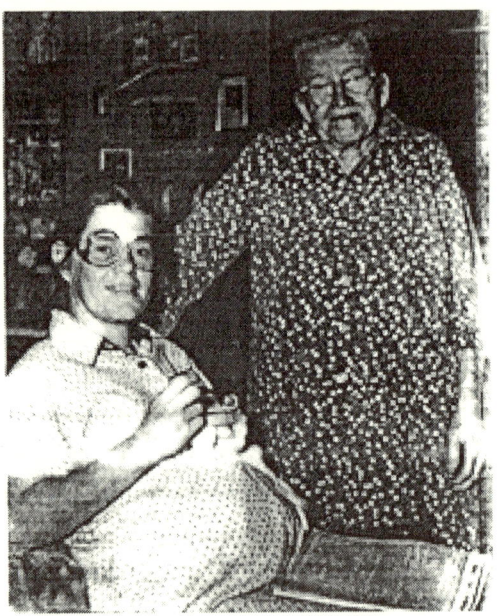

Mrs. Hamilton, seated, and midwife Nichols

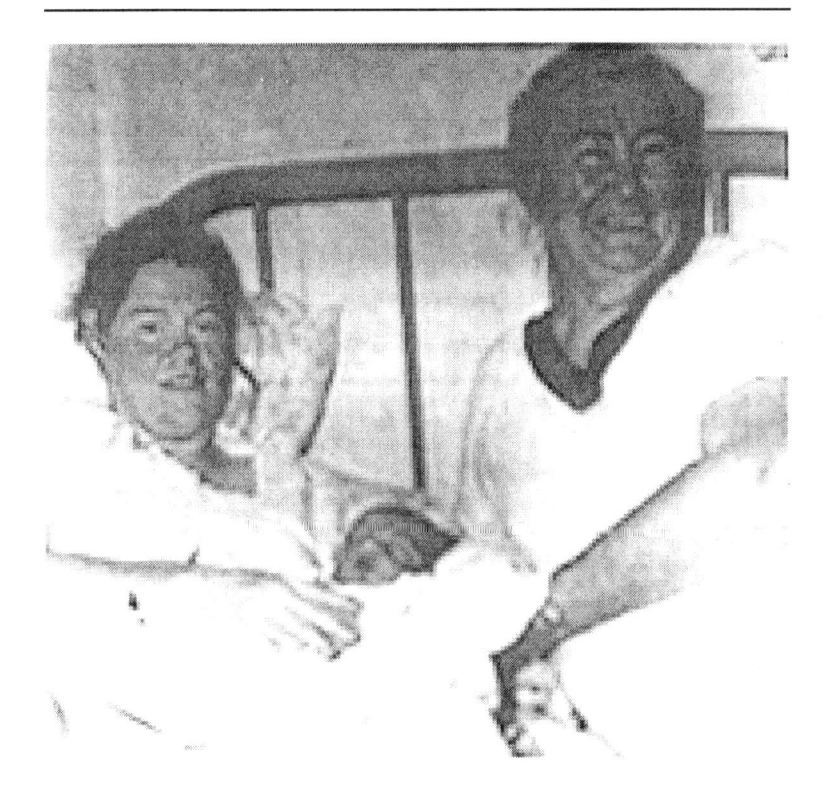

A 'beautiful' birth Tuesday

Midwife Etta Nichols, 86, of Del Rio witnessed another miracle of birth which she assisted Tuesday about noon. Giving birth to a seven pound girl was Mrs. Larry Hamilton, who has been in the news because she and her husband Rev. Hamilton had refused medical treatment for their daughter, Pamela, who is suffering with cancer. Mrs. Hamilton's mother, Lillian Crider, right, of Amarillo, Texas was in Cocke County to witness the birth of her 12th grandchild and called it a "beautiful birth." Rev. Hamilton is in Dalton, Georgia attending the Church of God Union Assembly, Inc. annual conference **(Photo by Shirley Elliott)**

News article and photos courtesy of The Newport Plain Talk.

During a visit Venida made to her grandparents, Etta was trying to get Harrison to dig her a hole in the corner of the yard so she could plant some flowers. Harrison procrastinated, saying he would do it later. Etta stomped out the back door and retrieved the mattock from the smoke house, then she walked to the site where she wanted the hole dug and began chopping at the ground. The mattock was about more than Etta could handle.

Harrison sat in his brown leather rocking chair staring out the window at Etta. After watching her for some time, Harrison turned to Venida, who was standing behind him, and said, "Doc's got more ambition than strength."

Venida laughed at her grandfather's dry humor. Eventually, Etta got the hole dug and a new, beautiful flower garden became part of the landscape.

• • • • • •

Sunday, November 20, 1983, started out just like any other day. After breakfast Harrison fed the goats, while Etta milked them. After the milking was done Harrison went to the fireplace to shovel out the ashes. Etta was in the kitchen when she heard a noise coming from the living room. She went quickly to see what was wrong. Harrison was holding on to the mantel and gasping for his breath. As Etta reached for him, Harrison started falling. Etta helped him to the floor. Harrison took his last breath in his wife's arms. He had experienced a massive heart attack. Harrison did not suffer, his death was almost instant. Etta could not believe what was happening. She ran to the telephone and called her son, Jack, for help, then she called Belle. Jack hurried over to his parents' house. When he walked into the living room he saw his father lying dead on the floor in front of the fireplace. Venida arrived with her mother, Belle, shortly after. Jack met Belle at the door and told her, "He's already gone."

Maloy's Funeral Home was notified, and they arrived shortly afterward to take Harrison to Newport where he would be prepared for burial, then they would bring him back to Etta's house for the funeral service.

Other family members and friends were notified about the passing of their loved one. Soon Etta's house was filled with people bringing food, and offering their sympathy, and their help. The family received friends for two nights. The funeral service was held on Tuesday with Rev. Darrell Allen and Rev. Dennis Caldwell officiating. Etta sat on the couch crying as she said good-bye to her beloved husband. They had celebrated their 67th wedding anniversary only one month previously, and now he was gone. Etta's heartbreak was almost unbearable. It saddened everyone to see Etta in so much pain, but the only thing anyone could do was to pray that God would help her get through her loss...and He did.

James Harrison Nichols died at the age of 87 on November 20, 1983. He was laid to rest in the Jonestown Cemetery on Highway 107 in Del Rio.

After Harrison's death Belle tried to persuade Etta to come live with her, but Etta would not hear of it, she was going to continue living at her own home, alone.

Several months passed until one day while Etta was at home by herself a strange man staggered up Etta's front steps and knocked on her door. Etta never did keep her doors locked during the daytime. When she went to the door she knew there was something wrong with this person from the very beginning. "What can I do for you?" Etta asked as she stepped out on the porch.

"I'm from the Social Security office. I need you to get out all your money and count it for me so I can report how much you keep on hand to the office," the stranger replied.

Etta stepped back inside and locked the screen door. The stranger tried to follow her in, but Etta turned around and told him firmly. "You stay right there!" She knew Harrison kept a .22 pistol in the house, so she went and got it and laid it on the bed, then she phoned the sheriff. The stranger must have seen her get the gun because when she looked out he was gone. Normally, it would take at least 20 minutes for an officer to reach Del Rio coming from Newport, but God must have been with Etta this day because there just happened to be an officer already in Del Rio answering another call. He was at Etta's house in a matter of minutes. Etta told the officer what the man had wanted her to do, and gave him a description.

The officer noticed the gun lying on Etta's bed. He said, "Well, I see you do have some protection."

"Yes, and I'll use it if I have to," Etta answered.

The officer left to go look for the man. Etta never did hear if the man was found or not. Nevertheless, she still did not lock her doors during the day. Her home was open to anyone who wanted to visit with her.

Etta "Granny" Nichols—Last of the Old-Timey Midwives

At 3:30 A.M. on the morning of April 18, 1984. Lloyd Manning from Newport knocked on Etta's door. He had brought his wife, Rebecca, to give birth. Etta showed Rebecca to the baby room and showed her where to lie down. Rebecca was already in hard labor. Lloyd paced the floor in the kitchen. Almost two hours later, at 5:27 A.M., Rebecca gave birth to a 7 pound baby girl. Rebecca and Lloyd named her Amanda Leanne Manning.

"Now, you two are goin' to have to eat some breakfast with me. You have to keep up your strength so you can take care of this little one," Etta told Lloyd and Rebecca.

Lloyd and Rebecca accepted Etta's invitation. Rebecca ate her breakfast in bed while she listened to Etta tell stories about her goats, and her family. Rebecca rested for about 30 minutes, then she was ready to get up and go home.

"Would you all like to take some apple pies home with you? I can put some foil over 'em, and put 'em in a poke for you," Etta offered.

"No, thanks, Mrs. Nichols. You have already done enough for us. You've been just wonderful. Thank you so much!" Rebecca answered as she prepared to leave.

"Well, I'm glad to do it. If you ever know of anybody goin' to have triplets, send 'em my way. I've delivered a bunch of twins, but I ain't been blessed with deliverin' triplets yet."

"We sure will," Lloyd said as he handed Etta her fee of $15. The happy couple smiled joyfully as they walked down the porch steps and got in their car with their new little baby girl.

• • • • • •

In the Summer of 1984 reporter Patricia A. Paquette from The Associated Press arrived at Etta's house to interview her for the newspaper where she worked. Her article said basically the same thing all the others did...how Etta became a midwife, the description of her birthing room, etc. One thing Patricia mentioned in her article that the others did not was the fact that expectant mothers and members of their family could stay with Etta as long as necessary, eat, and have their laundry done at no extra charge.

Also, in the Summer of 1984, Edie Ellis from NBC Channel 10 News, did an interview with Etta for "The Heartland Series". This series tells about special people and places in East Tennessee. Each episode lasts about ten minutes and airs after the morning and noonday news. Etta appeared on Episode XXV "Midwife".

On July 22, 1984, Etta received the sad news that her brother, Waitsel, had passed away. Etta was very close to Waitsel growing up, with him being the next-born child after herself. She would surely have yet another empty place in her heart.

Waitsel's funeral was held at Brown's Funeral Home in Newport. He was laid to rest at Clark Cemetery on Midway Road in Del Rio.

Etta became interested in keeping goats several years prior to 1984 when her sister, Alvertie Taylor, asked Etta to take some of her goats. Alvertie was moving into a house trailer down the road from Floyd and Belle, and she did not have enough room to keep her goats there, so Etta agreed to take them.

One evening in the Fall of 1984, Etta started to the field to milk the goats. As she walked up the trail leading to the barn, suddenly one of the goats ran towards her, butting her with its head very hard. When Etta fell to the ground she hit her head on a rock and broke three ribs. Etta lay unconscious on the ground for some time. With the help of the good Lord, Etta got herself up and made it back to the house to call for help. Belle went to tend to her mother right away. Belle helped Etta wrap some strands of old sheets around her waist and pulled them as tight as Etta could stand. After returning from the doctor's office, Etta had to go to bed and stay there until her ribs healed. Belle stayed with Etta while she was incapacitated. All of Etta's children tried to talk her into selling her goats after this terrible incident, but Etta refused. She was not getting rid of the goats!

Etta's grandson, Darrell Jones, came up from Morristown to help tend to Etta's goats and other chores outside while Etta recuperated. Everyone thought Etta would be immobilized for months, but she surprised them by only staying in bed a little over one week. She was not the kind of person to be in bed and let others wait on her. Etta's children worried that she was doing too much too soon, but she got around just fine. She had to turn away four expectant mothers while she was ill. Realizing how much she was needed gave her the strength to get up and get at it.

After Etta was well and back on her feet, Jerry Kirk arrived to do a story about Etta to print in the Tennessee

Sharon Smith-Ledford

<u>Cooperator Magazine</u>. The following article appeared in the next month's edition:

She's a loving living legend

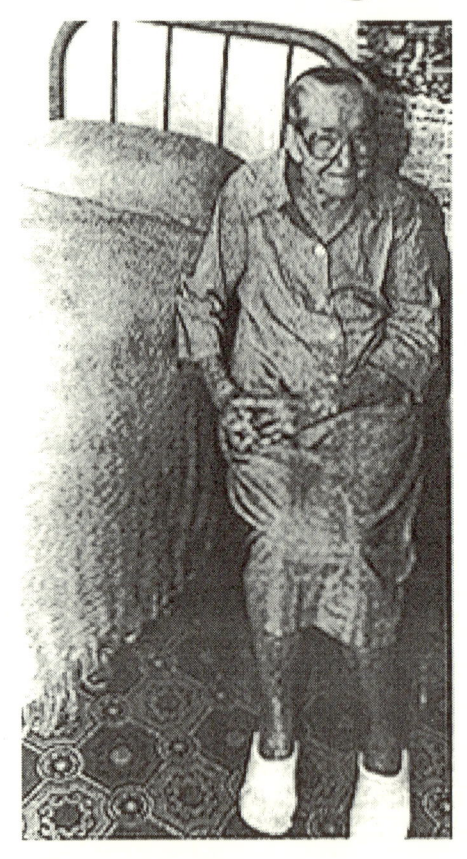

Story and photos by editor Jerry Kirk

Because Mrs. Etta Nichols had been feeling poorly, a neighbor stopped by to see if her goats needed milking.

Then, a son-in-law came by with a cabinet he had built for her kitchen.

Next came friends to buy some goat milk.

Within the span of about an hour on a pleasant fall morning, several people had driven the winding, scenic Cocke County road to the mountain home of 87-year-old Mrs. Nichols— more or less to check on "Miss Etta.

"It's like this all the time," said Mrs. Belle Smith, Mrs. Nichols' youngest daughter who was staying with her mother until Mrs. Nichols could get "back on her feet."

"Mamaw is a legend in these hills," said Darrell Jones, an employee of Hamblen Farmers Cooperative in Morristown and one of Mrs. Nichols' nine living grandchildren. "That's why people are always looking out after her."

Many folks have a special reason for showing such a loving interest in this soft-spoken, easy-going Christian lady. Those are the ones she delivered when they were born.

Mrs. Nichols has delivered more than 2,000 babies in nearly 55 years as a midwife. And she's still delivering them!

Family members emphasize, however, that because Mrs. Nichols' health isn't as good as it once was, she has had to cut back drastically on her midwifery.

"Why, I had to turn four down the week I got sick," Mrs. Nichols said, referring to her recent illness. "I couldn't get one of my feet off the floor...I just had to drag it. Never had such a hurting in my life."

She quickly turned her attention away from her ailments, though, to talk about her career as a midwife.

"I don't know exactly how many babies I've delivered, but it's something over 2,000," Mrs. Nichols said as she settled into her favorite chair in the "front room" of her spic-and-span house.

"She stopped counting a long time ago," daughter Belle replied.

The last full count was made in 1970, and the total at that time stood at 1,668 babies, according to Mrs. Nichols.

"We've got records on all the babies I've delivered, and I'm going to get them out one of these days and count them up," she promised, adding that her most recent delivery had been accomplished about three weeks earlier.

In her younger days, Mrs. Nichols would go to the homes of the expectant mothers to deliver the babies. In recent years, however, the mothers have come to her—to have their babies in a special "baby room" which Mrs. Nichols set up in her own home. The room has two beds, toilet facilities, scales, and other equipment.

Mrs. Nichols figures she must have come by her talents as a midwife naturally, considering the fact that her father, John Lewis Grigsby, was a doctor, as was his father.

"My father told me a lot, especially on how to take care of the mother and baby both after the baby was born, Mrs. Nichols said.

She hadn't had the benefit of instruction from her father, though, when she was called on to deliver her first baby 54 years ago.

That first delivery came at the home of a woman who lived right in above us in the Blue Mill area of Cocke County, Mrs. Nichols recalled.

"They had gone after my father to come and deliver the baby, but he was gone and nobody knew where he was," she explained. "The woman's brother asked me if I would go and I did. I delivered that baby without any problems."

"Next thing I knew, somebody else sent for me...and then somebody else," Mrs. Nichols added. "Then, I delivered a set of twins for another woman. I've been going ever since."

Mrs. Nichols was about 33 years old when she delivered the first baby. Since then, she's delivered babies "all over Cocke County, over in North Carolina—as far away as Marshall—and all the way down to Douglas Dam (in Jefferson County, Tenn.)."

"I've delivered around 20 sets of twins, but so far I haven't delivered any triplets," she said. "I'm hoping the Lord will let me live long enough to do that."

Mrs. Nichols can remember wading snow "halfway to my knees" as she made house calls to deliver babies.

"We didn't have a car, so it was either walk or ride horseback or go in a wagon or buggy," she said. When she had to go over into North Carolina, folks would come and get her, "mostly in trucks."

"I used to would rather ride in a truck as in a car," Mrs. Nichols said. "For some reason, I would get as sick as a buzzard in a car."

She had her own little black bag that she carried with her when she "went out" to deliver her babies.

And she always carried with her the most important thing she thinks a midwife can have. That's patience. "You can't be nervous and you've got to have confidence and know what you're doing," she said.

Mrs. Nichols said it seems that more babies are born between the hours of 5 and 7 in the morning, but she has no thoughts on why that is.

A birth certificate is filled out on each baby delivered by Mrs. Nichols, and the information is filed with the state. The mother is given a copy of the birth certificate.

Mrs. Nichols has delivered several of her own grandchildren, including Co-op employee Jones.

"Yes, I was born right back there in that room," Darrell said, pointing to the special baby room.

Some of the babies Mrs. Nichols has delivered are now grandparents themselves.

"Oh, I've tried to keep up with all the babies, but I just can't do it...there's too many of them," Mrs. Nichols said. "Some of them, I'm sorry to say, I don't even recognize when I see them. They'll say to me, "Why, you delivered me!"

When women arrive at Mrs. Nichols' house—perched in a picturesque spot in the hills above Del Rio—to have their babies, they know they're going to experience natural childbirth.

"There's no doping up of the mothers here," Mrs. Nichols said, adding proudly that she has never had to call a doctor in to help with a delivery.

Usually, a mother who has her baby in the morning in Mrs. Nichols' baby room is able to go home "along down in the evening."

"I just can't keep the women in the bed but a little while," the midwife said. "They tell me they feel good and want to get up. It's very seldom that I have to take more than one meal to the bed to them. They'll come out to the kitchen table to eat."

While Mrs. Nichols has spent most of her life in the Cocke County hills where she was born, her fame as a midwife has become more widespread—thanks to television and the printed word.

She has been the subject of various articles in newspapers and magazines and featured in books. She's been on television four or five times.

"I've had letters from people 'way off from here that say they've read about me in the paper," she said. "I just can't imagine why anybody would want to read about me, though I never did take a good picture, and I don't think I look good on TV."

Of course, those are just her opinions. Others find her story fascinating—and they enjoy seeing what she looks like.

Mrs. Nichols has been a widow for more than a year now. Her husband, James Harrison Nichols, died on Thanksgiving Day of 1983. Mr. and Mrs. Nichols had four children, and three are still living. Jones' mother, Mrs. Emily Nichols Jones, is deceased. Daughter Belle and the Nichols' only son, Jack, live near their mother. The other daughter, Mrs. June Gilliland, lives in Morristown.

Mrs. Nichols enjoys the times any of her nine grandchildren, 23 great-grandchildren, or two great-great-grandchildren can visit.

She enjoys, too, taking care of her 13 goats, three of which are currently being milked. Somebody else comes in now to do the milking, but Mrs. Nichols still likes the milk.

"It's the best buttermilk you'll ever drink," she said.

She'll keep her baby room open as long as she can, too, even though she won't be able to perform the number of deliveries she once could.

Medical personnel in the area have never tried to interfere with Mrs. Nichols' midwifery.

"They know not to," daughter Belle said. "There are too many people around here who know and love her."

"People in these hills would take up for her...I know they would," grandson Jones said.

"Why, there'd be a war if anybody tried to do anything to keep her from delivering babies," Belle predicted.

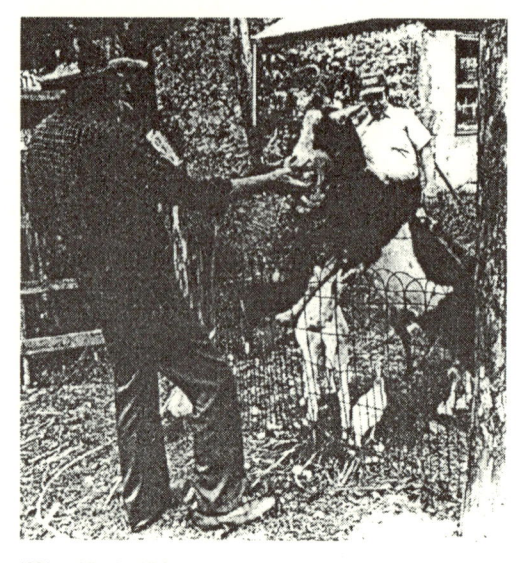

1984—While Mrs. Nichols recuperates from a recent illness, a son-in-law, John Gilliland, left, and a grandson, Darrell Jones, a member of the Hamblen Farmers Co-op staff see to her goats.

Article and photos courtesy of the Tennessee Cooperator.

On Sunday, September 8, 1985, The Atlanta Journal and Constitution ran a special interview with Etta in that paper. Tom Eblen was the staff writer, and Gary Hamilton was the photographer.

On a Monday night in October, 1985, Etta appeared on the NBC Nightly News with Tom Brokaw. The Newport Plain Talk sent reporter Shirley Elliott to cover the story.

NBC crew at Del Rio to film midwife, child

By Shirley Elliott

Mrs. Nichols, a legend and the last of her kind, has practiced midwifery for 55 years in the mountains of Del Rio.

At age 88 her pace may have slowed, but not her spirit and her love for her work, delivering babies.

She has delivered well over 2,000 babies including 20 sets of twins during her career.

For the past 25 years she has delivered her babies in the labor-delivery room at her home which is a 9 foot square room with two beds, a toilet, sink and two medicine cabinets. The room was added on to the house when she was no longer able to make house calls.

The NBC crew had been to the Nichols' home several weeks ago and finished filming the first part of their story. A midwife story would not be complete without filming a birth, so when Wanda McCarter of Route 1, Cosby, called and said she was on her way, the crew in Atlanta, Ga., also received a call. They were soon on their way to Del Rio. Peggy Sue, an eight and one-half pound girl arrived at about the time the crew arrived at the home. The filming was almost completed by 2:30 A.M. Wednesday, October 9. A return to the home Wednesday afternoon for an interview with Mrs. McCarter and for another look at Peggy Sue wrapped up their story which will hopefully be aired at 6:30 P.M. on the NBC Nightly News with Tom Brokaw, Friday (tonight), October 11. Kenley Jones will be reporting the TV story.

The crew who came to Del Rio this week included the sound man, Cecil O'Neil, cameraman, Jeff Klein, and interviewer, Donna Mastrangelo.

Mrs. Mastrangelo said if it did not appear Friday night to watch next week and it would be on one night.

Wanda and James Stanley McCarter are the parents of three other children, Dale, age 12, Sheila, age 4, and James, age 2. They were all delivered by "Granny Nichols," as she is fondly called by patients. Mrs. McCarter said, "Having a baby without Granny just wouldn't be the. same.

The charge for a delivery is $15.00, "but they usually give me a little more," the midwife said.

A group of Del Rio citizens have banded together and hope to build the "Etta Nichols Clinic" in Del Rio in the future. "If they charge too much, they can just take my name off," Mrs. Nichols said.

She once said, "If they can't pay, I don't push them. I don't want one of these babies going hungry."

If things go as planned, a reporter from National Geographic will be present for her next delivery scheduled in about three weeks.

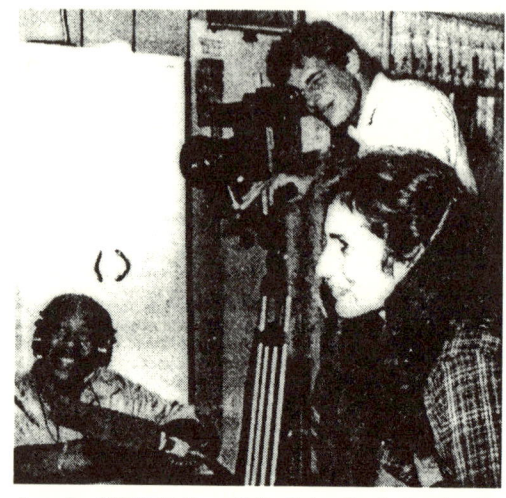

A crew from NBC Nightly News with Tom Brokaw filmed a story about Mrs. Etta Nichols, Del Rio midwife. From left are Cecil O'Neil, Jeff Klein, and Donna Mastrangelo. The story is being aired tonight (Friday, October 11) at 6:30 P.M. **(photo by Shirley Elliott)**

News article and photos courtesy of The Newport Plain Talk.

Etta's children and grandchildren watched Etta on the news proudly that night, knowing their loved one was being seen by an entire nation of people. The event was recorded on a VCR along with the episode of Etta's appearance on "The Heartland Series." This definitely was a treasure for the entire family to pass down through the generations to come. When Sharon showed Etta the tape of herself on television she just turned red-faced as her body shook in laughter.

Etta was not used to watching television. She had never owned one while Harrison was alive. He said television was the devil's toy, and would not allow one in the house. After Harrison's death, one of Etta's patients paid her by giving her a 19-inch black and white television. Etta hardly ever turned it on, although she did enjoy watching the news and "The Price Is Right." It came in handy for Etta's patients, too. Before she got the television the women had nothing to do with their time, now at least they had some entertainment until they went into hard labor.

Michael Sylva had entered a photograph of Harrison and Etta, with a quilt pattern for the border of the photograph, in a contest for the pictures that would appear in the 1986 Tennessee Homecoming Calendar. Michael's photograph of Harrison and Etta won a prize, and the photograph appeared in the calendar for the month of January.

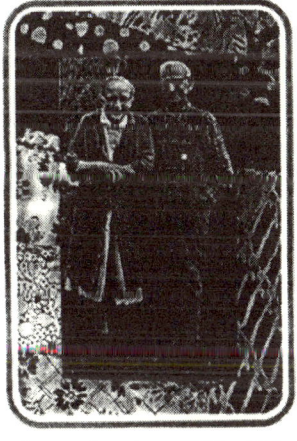

photograph courtesy of Michael Sylva

In January, 1986, Etta once again appeared in <u>The Newport Plain Talk</u> newspaper, and again in March of that year.

Etta would soon turn 89 years old, on May 19, 1986. A friend of hers, Susanna Lane, stayed with Etta during the day sometimes to help out with the chores around the house. Susanna and her daughter rented the house in London where Etta's mother had lived before Harrison died. Now Susanna lived in Newport. Susanna was a nurse so she also helped Etta check her patients when Etta needed her to. The two women seemed to enjoy one another's company very much. They both enjoyed the same things in life.

Susanna was fighting a bout of cancer, and her health was steadily declining. On April 18, 1986, Susanna suffered a fatal heart attack. She was buried in Ray's Chapel Cemetery in Newport. Etta certainly would miss her beloved friend.

In the April edition of *People* Magazine, Etta tells her story on pages 59 through 63. This was probably one of the best interviews Etta had done so far, as far as covering a lot of different information about her life.

Also in April, 1986, <u>The Newport Plain Talk</u> printed the following article:

Etta "Granny" Nichols—Last of the Old-Timey Midwives

OUR VIEWPOINT

She was born to serve and deserves recognition

Sometimes you can go through life without noticing those rare individuals in your own community who have never been recognized for their outstanding achievements.

One such person who has built an incredible monument to life by helping thousands of people and perpetuating our mountain heritage is Etta Nichols of Del Rio. Affectionately known as Granny Nichols, she has been responsible for bringing into this world over 2,000 babies as a midwife. She has not lost one infant at birth.

She got some much deserved publicity in the April issue of "People" magazine in which she told her story to millions of readers. It is a story of love and understanding but especially of dedication to helping and serving others and to a determination to perpetuate the human touch.

A mother, grandmother, great or great, great greandmother to 26 she spreads her loving touch over the mountains and imparts the message that people make a difference. She makes no pretensions about being a healer, great leader, intellectual or celebrity. She's a mountain woman, proud of her heritage and wise in ways that have meant life to thousands.

The county has never given her the recognition she deserves. Perhaps during Homecoming '86 she will be singled out as exemplifying many of the good and beautiful traits of our people. We could think of no better person to welcome home people born here.

We appreciate you, Granny Nichols. Thanks for being there when mothers needed you.

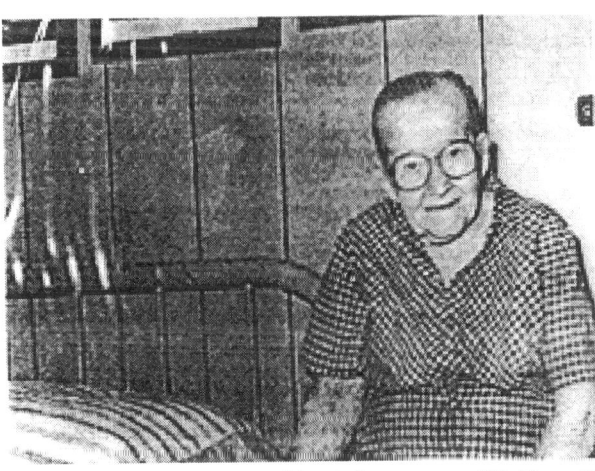

NEWPORT PLAIN TALK, Friday, April 4, 1986

News article and photos courtesy of The Newport Plain Talk

In the May 1986, issue of <u>National Geographic</u> magazine, Vol. 169, No. 5, Etta appeared on page 629, and there was also an article in *STAR* about her.

It seemed there was a reporter wanting to interview Etta every month or so now, but Etta did not let it go to her head. She remained the same down-to-earth, loving person she had always been. If she wanted to go barefooted while the reporters were there, she did. She did not put on any pretenses for anyone.

Belle went over to help her mother every chance she could, but having her own family to care for was putting too much stress on Belle, and June lived too far away to come down every day. Etta agreed to find a live-in female companion to stay with her to help lighten Belle's load; Etta still would not leave her home to move in with Belle, or June. After talking to several women in the community, Hassa Lee Raines was chosen to be Etta's companion. She was a good person and Etta's children knew they could count on her to take good care of their mother.

On August 1, 1986, Etta received word that her son-in-law, Dick Jones, had died from a heart attack. He was laid to rest in the Jarnigan Cemetery in Morristown.

In October 1986, Governor Lamar Alexander honored Etta by giving her a Tennessee Homecoming certificate signed by him, and a state flag that had flown in Nashville. Harold Cates presented the honors to Etta in her home. The following article in <u>The Newport Plain Talk</u> covered the event:

Etta "Granny" Nichols—Last of the Old-Timey Midwives

Gov. Alexander honors midwife Nichols

By Nancy Oberst

Lamar Alexander has never met the Del Rio woman people call "Granny Nichols," but the governor signed a certificate saying she's special to Tennessee's heritage.

Harold Cates met her about 25 years ago, and he was scared to death because he went to bring midwife Etta Nichols to a mother who was having a baby, he thought, right then. He knew one tiny thing about birthing babies: Go get Granny Nichols.

Since then, the director of human services in Cocke County has brought mothers to the mid-wife and he's given directions to her home to other mothers who couldn't afford to have their babies delivered at a hospital. Twenty-five years after his first meeting, Cates went to the mid-wife's home to deliver a piece of paper and a flag.

The piece of paper is a Tennessee Homecoming '86 certificate, signifying Etta Nichols is an important part of the state's heritage. The flag is a state flag that has billowed over the capitol building in Nashville.

Cates was dead-set on having Department of Human Services Commissioner Marguerite

One of these days she will quit, "when my toes are sticking up."

Sallee present the certificate and flag to Nichols at the open-house of the new DHS office on October 2. The 89-year-old midwife's legs have been bothering her, so she couldn't come to town.

"I couldn't get you to town, so I thought I'd take it to you," he told her.

One of these days she will quit, "when my toes are sticking up."

What does she think about all the fuss made over her by people like the governor? "I'd rather people say good things as bad."

After receiving the certificate and flag, she said, "I don't think I deserve them."

Cates said, "that's why I think you do."

About their first meeting when the 25-years-younger pair met: "I hadn't been the director long and I got this anonymous call late one night from a man about a person having a baby and they couldn't get a doctor." The young mother already had two small children and when Cates found her home in Newport, he saw "it was a real shack with no electricity or indoor plumbing.

"The children were crying and scared and the mother was scared." If the truth is told, he was scared, too.

"She couldn't find a doctor to deliver her baby. I had heard of Etta Nichols in Del Rio, but I had never met her." The midwife was the only solution he could find.

So he took the children to one of the mother's neighbors and went to get the midwife. He didn't even know where Nichols lived, just somewhere in Del Rio. He had to get her

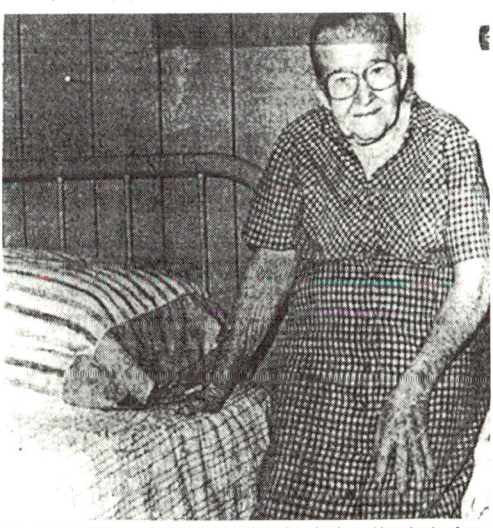

Etta Nichols is in her birthing room where hundreds and hundreds of area people were born. Above the other iron post bed is a portrait of Mrs. Nichols and her late husband, James Harrison Nichols, photographed b Michael Sylva, of Del Rio. The photograph is included in the Tennessee Homecoming '86 calendar. (photo by Nancy Oberst)

211

Sharon Smith-Ledford

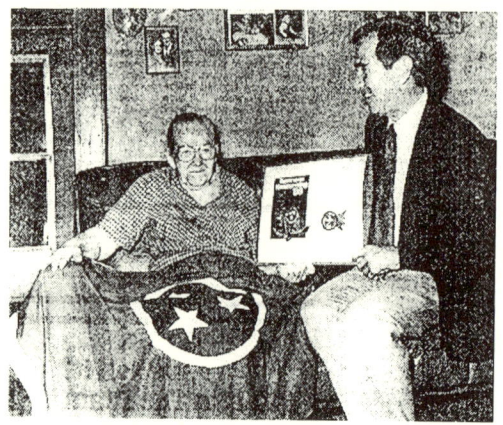

Honored in her home for decades of service to Cocke County with her midwifery skills, Etta Nichols receives a Tennessee Homecoming '86 certificate signed by Governor Lamar Alexander and a state flag that has flown in Nashville. Cocke County Department of Human Services Director Harold Cates presented the honors to Etta Nichols last week at her Del Rio home. (photo by Nancy Oberst)

himself because she didn't have a phone then.

By then that night it was about 11 o'clock and he knocked on doors until he found the midwife's house, where she still lives and where she's lived nearly 50 years. She and her Chihuahuas, cats, chickens, and goats live beyond where Highway 107 forks one way to Round Mountain and the other way to her place.

There was a little obstacle in front of Cates that night. A footlog.

"I could see everything happening to me," including falling in the creek. So he shined his headlight' on the path. That didn't do much good, but neither did he fall in. There isn't a footlog anymore; there's a regular graveled driveway over a tile.

He told Nichols who he was and what he wanted. In a few minutes "she came to the door with a little black bag and said, 'I'm ready,'" Cates said.

When they arrived at the woman's coarse house, he and a neighbor "had to fix hot water; we had to build a fire. I don't know what she needed hot water for." He still doesn't know a lot about birthing babies. At least his son does; Hal is Dr. Cates now and he's a resident practicing in Kentucky.'

Nichols told Cates to go on home because it would be a while before the baby would come. Relieved he went home.

"That was my introduction to one of the most fabulous ladies I've ever known," Cates said.

With the occasion of Cates bringing her Governor Alexander's message, she said, "I can't hardly tell you how I feel. I just think it's alright."

She's been famous in her own Cocke County for years - she's been featured in the Newport Plain Talk several times through the decades. Her midwifery training was at the side of her father, who was a country doctor, and she has been delivering babies about half a century.

Lately the unassuming woman's face has become known everywhere the photographs of her in the National Geographic and People have been seen. She has also been featured on the NBC Nightly News.

How does she feel about everyone's interest in her?

"I've not asked, none of them. It don't make me mad; I appreciate it."

It doesn't even bother her that she's never made hardly any money delivering babies. "I haven't counted them up since '70; I'm going to do that soon," she said. In 1970, the babies totaled about 1,600 so she figures she has delivered at least 400 more since then. Those babies include several sets of twins, and her biggest ambition is to deliver triplets.

She and her late husband, James Harrison Nichols, had four children themselves.

The most the midwife ever charged is $15. The fee used to he three or four dollars, "just sort of what they were able to pay. I've delivered eight and nine for a family and never got a bit out of them," she said with a crinkled smile.

But there is one little thing that does get her ire up. "Every now and then the news gets out that I've quit delivering, but I haven't." She delivered a baby on September 16 and "there's never a week passes that I have to check a woman."

One of these days she will quit, "when my toes are sticking up."

News article and photos courtesy of The Newport Plain Talk.

Etta "Granny" Nichols—Last of the Old-Timey Midwives

On Saturday, November 15, 1986, The Greeneville Sun, in Greeneville, Tennessee, featured the following article written by Bob Hurley in their paper:

Delivering Babies More Than Just A Job For Famed Midwife

By BOB HURLEY
Sun Columnist

She is a tiny lady, almost miniature compared to some of the rest of us. Her dress is long, almost to her ankles. Her hair is silver and pulled tightly back into an old-style granny knot on the back of her head.

Her back is stooped, her steps slowed by her 89 years and some old problems with her feet and legs. Part of a toe is missing from an accident long ago, and her legs are red and sore-looking, a problem she has battled for a long time and still battles every day. The only unmistakable part of her appearance that rings of 1986 is the mod glasses that sit on her nose.

But her eyes still twinkle when she giggles, and even at 89, she still giggles. A lot. She has never been known as the giggling granny of Del Rio, but Etta Nichols can burst into the kind of contagious laughter that spreads through her little part of the world like wildfire.

To her neighbors, she is Granny Nichols, a midwife in a fading tradition of the Cocke County mountains she calls home. For close to 60 years, her job has been to deliver babies and care for new mothers in a way all but forgotten outside these mountains.

But it is much more than just a job. It is more like a calling to her, a little like missionary work that has led her through a full and active life, one where she says she counts "the blessings of the Lord while serving my people." She has also won the blessings of neighboring physicians, some of whom send expectant mothers to her for the delivery.

She has come to be known as the first lady of Del Rio, a title she wears well, perhaps from her gentle nature and the motherly image she projects while wearing her home-make aprons and talking her homespun ways.

Etter, as she's also known around Del Rio, is one of a handful of granny-type midwives, a holdover, it seems, from another time. She still delivers babies in much the same way her father did. He doctored the sick and delivered several generations of Del Rio babies during his career that stretched back to the Civil War.

She wanted to be a nurse, but there was no money for schooling and not enough time, either. The horseback, door-to-door practice of her father was also a missionary-type career. There were not many rich doctors at Del Rio when Etter was a girl.

Meeting the medical needs of people ran in the family. Her grandfather was also a doctor.

So it was only natural that she dreamed of being a nurse. When circumstances made that impossible, it was only natural that she become a midwife.

"Doctors have always been scarce around here," she said, standing in the shadows of Round Mountain earlier in the fall, back when the weather was more summery than this.

"The doctors have always had more than they could get done, so midwives have been necessary to meet a need, a need that's as natural as can be."

The little home sits beside Ground Squirrel Road, which is the last one before the logging roads start. The home is also her office, delivery room, maternity ward and visitor center.

It is the visitor center part that I am now most familiar with. Actually, it is her well-worn front porch that I have come to love. I've spent a lot of time with her there. I first came here well over a year ago.

It would be great if I could say that I was the first to thrust Etter into the public eye. Far from that, I am just the latest in a very long string. She is practically a fixture on national television with appearances on "60 Minutes" and the "NBC Nightly News" to her recent credit. She has been in more national publications than she care to keep

213

up with, including People Magazine and a full page picture in a recent National Geographic that she didn't like, and she'd like to tell National Geographic that she didn't like it.

Now, Etter loves everybody. The Lord knows that. But newsmen have a way of getting on her nerves like you wouldn't believe. They have this certain air about them, Etter will tell you, that is not only a little pushy, but it is a little out of place on Ground Squirrel Road. It might be an acceptable way of getting things done in those big cities where TV anchormen smile from, but this is Del Rio. No smoking and no pushing are allowed in Etter's house.

Over the past year or so, I guess I've stopped by Etter's place close to a dozen times. I am just as amazed now as I was after that first visit.

I have taken my time with Etter and her story for a lot of reasons, but only two of them are important enough for you to know about her. One, I loved to be around her so much that I deliberately delayed the process as long as humanly possible, and, secondly, I kept waiting for the world's most beautiful baby to arrive here so I could get a picture of It with Etter.

The world's most beautiful baby came a few days back. Her name is Sara Tenille Sutton, five pounds and four ounces of pure joy. If you don't believe she is the world's most beautiful, just ask Joyce and Rick Sutton, the proud parents.

I'm convinced I did the right thing to wait, because Sara is indeed beautiful, her dark hair made darker and more shiny by the liberal amounts of baby oil that Etter massaged into it. I'm also convinced because Rick and Joyce are among Etter's biggest

and most loyal, most loving fans. They drove all the way from Nashville to Del Rio just so Etter could deliver Sara Tenille. That's more than five hours on the road with Joyce in such a motherly way that travel just wasn't much fun at all.

"Sara Tenille is the second of two children for us, both of them delivered by Mrs. Nichols," Rick said. "That's it. I'm going myself next week."

I think I know what that means.

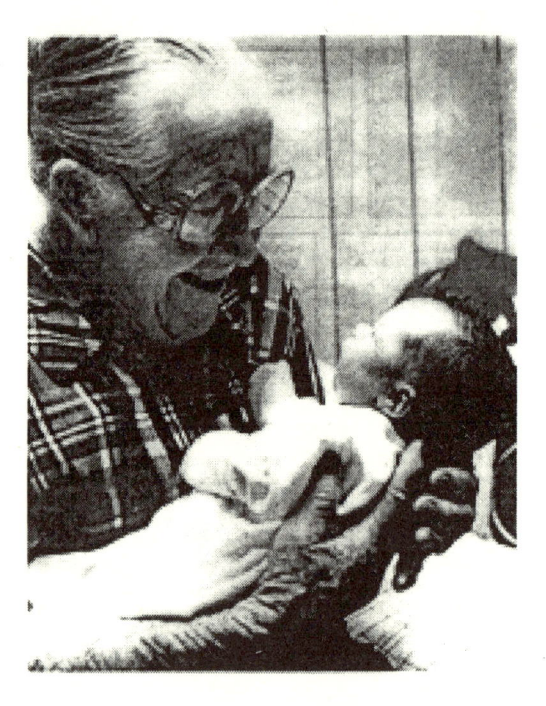

"We had a doctor for her prenatal care," he said, "but we can't get over how wonderful Mrs. Nichols is at the actual delivery. She tells us everything there is to know. And everything there is to do. She is amazing.

"Childbirth is not a disease or an illness as some people would have you think. It is a miracle of God," said Rick, who works, in Nashville, with the Rev. Jimmy Snow on the Gospel Country Network. Snow is the son of the legendary Hank Snow of the Grand Ole Opry and the County Music Hall of Fame.

Rick is the construction engineer for Jimmy Snow's Grand Old Gospel Show, which airs on Nashville's WSM Radio on Sunday nights.

It was Etta's national television exposure that brought the Suttons to Del Rio.

"We saw her first in national TV about mid way of Joyce's pregnancy with Christopher and we had already paid half of what was to be a $3,000 delivery fee in Nashville.' We forgot about the money and drove' up here to hunt Mrs. Nichols.

"Actually, I called the Chamber of Commerce in Newport first. They knew all about Mrs. Nichols and they told me how to get to Ground Squirrel Road. They even wanted to send me some brochures about her.

"I told them that wouldn't be necessary because I was leaving right then for Del Rio. We drove up here, found her, got to know her, loved her and told her we'd see her in around four months. When Christopher was due, we drove back up here and Joyce presented me with what you see here," he said, holding up a very bright-eyed Christopher Sutton.

If I was amazed at Etter and her ways, Rick was doubly amazed.

He loves the little lady so much that he'd like to take her home to Nashville with him.

Etter, however, is not leaving Ground Squirrel Road. She doesn't even go to town anymore. Her children and grandchildren bring in the groceries. She stays right here and milks her goats and delivers her babies.

And they are indeed her babies, more than 2,000 of them in the last 57 years. She claims them all.

"Now, you bring my baby back to see me," she ordered Rick and Joyce as they left to return to Nashville.

Times were hard back when she started delivering babies. She learned to get by with precious little. She never forgot. She still gets by with precious little. Her fee is as flexible as her schedule. If the baby wants to be born at three in the morning after a terrible night of agony on the mother's part, Etter will be there. If the father wants to pay $15 for the trouble, that will be all right. If he doesn't have the 15 bucks, that will be all right too.

Some, of course, pay her more.

"One daddy gave me a hundred dollars one time," she said, her eyes twinkling again.

"When I started, people didn't have enough money to live on, much less to pay a doctor. I'm here to serve the Lord and I do that by helping my people, pay or no pay. I figure a person has got to do what is set before you to do. When people need help, you've got to help. When you do your best to help people, I figure the Lord will see to it that your needs are met. He has always met mine.

"All in all, I've had a wonderful life. I had a wonderful husband (Harrison Nichols died three years ago), a wonderful family of children and grandchildren. And I've got over 2,000 babies out there that I love and many of them come to see me."

If you think she's kidding about the 2,000, think again. The times that I have been at her house have been just a little hard for me to believe. Here we are, smack in the middle of these mountains where the nearest country store is at least five miles back down the road, and it's like we were on Main Street at the rush hour. Folks come and go around here like this is indeed a place where babies are being born.

Three is the highest number of babies she remembers delivering in one day's time, and five is the most she remembers in any one week. Around Etter's place, deliveries are as common as milking time.

And all I wanted to do was to help with one of them. Or I thought I wanted to help. I told her that I had never observed a delivery and I was wondering if she would allow me to see how all this happens.

I shouldn't have asked her that, because it was then that I saw the other side of Granny Nichols, the fighting side. The twinkle in her eyes turned to a pierce.

"Young man, I'll have you know this is no cattle show I'm running here. We're dealing with human beings, precious little babies, made in the image of God and I'll quit this business before I open it up and make a show out of it.

"Now, you're welcome to stay as long as you like, right through supper and all, but when it comes time for babies to be born, there will be no man in my little room except the father of the baby if he wants to be, and if he can stand the sight of it.

"That television camera man that busted in there after one of my babies had been born a couple of years ago would have gotten thrown out of here on his head if I hadn't been so busy and all. That man is no longer welcome here. Babies and their mothers are serious business. Can't people see that?"

After she stopped preaching my funeral, I didn't ask her any more silly questions. I just sort of hung around to see what would happen next. What happened was Sara Tenille, the beauty.

It all seemed so natural. One hour, Joyce was sitting here talking to us. The next hour, she's in there having a baby. The next morning, she's back up; filling out her baby's birth certificate and getting ready to head back to Nashville.

I felt like an eyewitness to nature, and I had never felt that way before. I may never get to feel that way again.

It was time to leave. Etter and Joyce and Rick are so much like family that they laughed and cried and hugged all at the same time.

And I was down to just one problem: now that I've done her story, I have no good excuse to go sit on Etter's front porch. And I feel a little empty because of it.

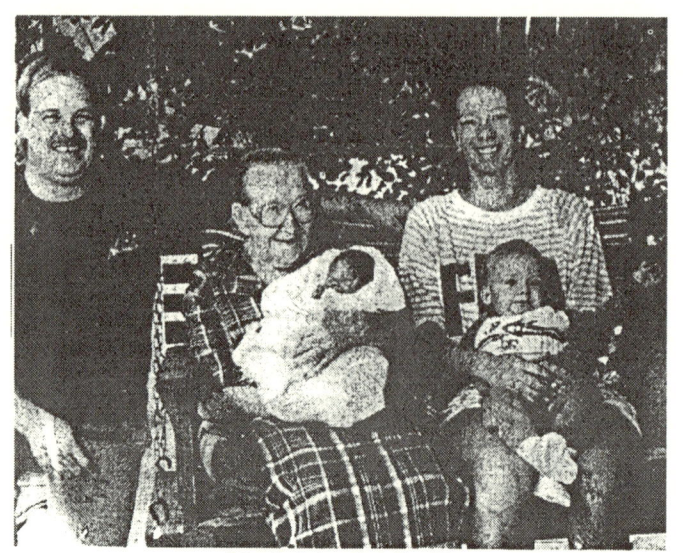

Sutton family from Nashville—'86

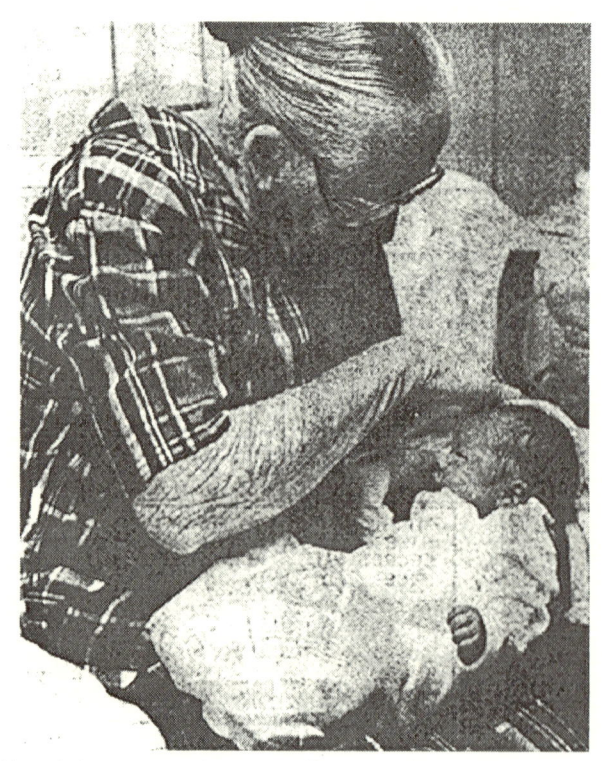

News articles and photos courtesy of The Greeneville Sun.

Etta "Granny" Nichols—Last of the Old-Timey Midwives

Etta would turn 90 years old on May 19, 1987. Her children and grandchildren celebrated the happy occasion on Mother's Day, May 10. David Popiel was there to record the event on film for The Newport Plain Talk. Also, the National Bank of Newport ran a special large ad wishing Etta a happy birthday. State Representative Ronnie Davis introduced a resolution to honor Etta's 90th, which also appeared in The Newport Plain Talk.

Birthdays are her specialty

David Popiel
Editor

She is well-acquainted with births. May 19 will bring her 90th birthday but she has been close at hand for thousands of others.

Margaret Carrie "Etta" Nichols will take another birthday in stride Tuesday, having been surprised Mother's Day weekend by dozens of her friends and children at her Del Rio home. Her three children are: Jack and Belle Smith, of Del Rio, and June Gilliland, of Morristown, and she has the memory of a fourth, Emile.

For 40 winters, Mrs. Nichols has lived on Ground Squirrel Road, which used to be Laurel Branch until the road was rebuilt and a neighbor observed a squirrel digging into it.

Until 1983 she lived with her husband, James Harrison Nichols, who suffered a stroke and died at home. But that didn't stop her work for which she has gained a national prominence. Since her 30s (about 60 years ago) she has been a midwife. By 1970, she had delivered more than 1,650 children and stopped counting. She suspects that more than 2,000 children received her welcome and the touch of her caring hands.

Born Margaret Carrie Grigsby not far from her present home near Blue Mill, she grew up much as any child raised in the mountains. She has been well-acquainted with work and has that knack to make anyone feel like a long-time friend. Sit on her porch a spell and talk—her eyes are full of the knowing wisdom of a mother of many children.

Her best advice to mothers: "Teach your children to do right." She could have offered a lot of health care advice, but she picks information that molds inner lives. And, experience teaches her that "doing right" is important. After all, she has 13 grandchildren, 28 great-grandchildren and two great-great-grandchildren.

While celebrating her birthday quietly among the pines, a brilliant white church steeple just down the gravel road, and a creek continuously talking in the spring air, she will be thinking about her children. "I call them all mine." Even on birthdays past, she has delivered children. At 90 she hasn't stopped, having delivered a child in February and expecting another in July "...or before. I never know when someone's going to come to my door."

Some of her own grandchildren felt the first touch of her soft hands. Many lives spin off from her warm presence, and she gets words and massages back and smiles. She has done a good work. What better gift on a birthday than to have a child named after you? Many Margaret Carrie Ettas will cherish her. The candles at her 90th are as bright as ever.

Representative Ronnie Davis introduced the following resolution to honor Cocke County midwife Mrs. James Harrison Nichols on her ninetieth birthday.

WHEREAS, Midwifery, the art and practice of attending women in childbirth, is a time honored tradition which dates from at least ancient Greece and Rome where it was an integral part of the social structure; and

WHEREAS, Midwifery continued to be an important

Sharon Smith-Ledford

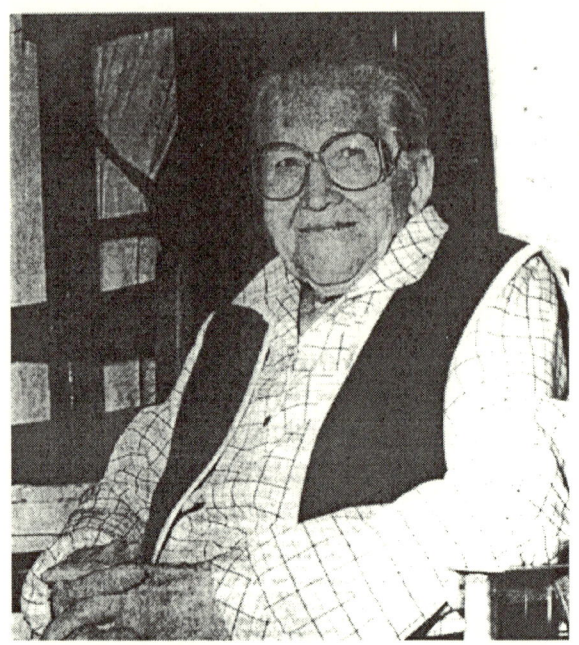

Margaret Carrie "Etta" Nichols, of Del Rio, takes her 90th birthday in stride, which she celebrates on May 19. She was surrounded by her children, grandchildren, and great-grandchildren on Sunday, May 10, for Mother's Day. (photo by David Popiel)

factor in births until the middle of the 20th century and is still practiced in many rural sections of Tennessee; and

WHEREAS, Mrs. James Harrison Nichols, a widely loved resident of Cocke County, has been a midwife for more than 55 years, providing an inexpensive service for many who cannot afford a hospital birth; and

WHEREAS, Mrs. Nichols was raised with a medical background around her as both her grandfather, John B. Grigsby, and her father, J. L. Grigsby, were physicians; and

WHEREAS, She learned both how to perform child births and to care for her patients from accompanying her father on house calls; and

WHEREAS, Always desiring to make the birth process easier for the mother, Mrs. Harrison has prepared a special room where the mother can stay until she feels ready to go home; and

WHEREAS, She has delivered well over 2,000 babies including 20 sets of twins; and

WHEREAS, Because of her fine work, the National Broadcasting Company had a feature story about her on their widely watched Nightly News program; and

WHEREAS, The May 1988 National Geographic mentioned her as an excellent example of the value of midwives and quoted Etta in a characteristic manner as saying she "won't retire till my toes are sticking up;" and

WHEREAS, on May 19, 1987, she will celebrate her ninetieth birthday, a day that will be a joyous celebration of her lifetime of service to the Del Rio area; and

WHEREAS, It is appropriate that we pause to specially honor this woman who has meant so much to her community; now, therefore,

BE IT RESOLVED BY THE HOUSE OF REPRESENTATIVES OF THE NINETY-FIFTH GENERAL ASSEMBLY OF THE STATE OF TENNESSEE, That we honor and congratulate Mrs. James Harrison Nichols, whose youth and vitality should serve as an inspiration to all of us and wish her many happy returns on the celebration of her ninetieth birthday.

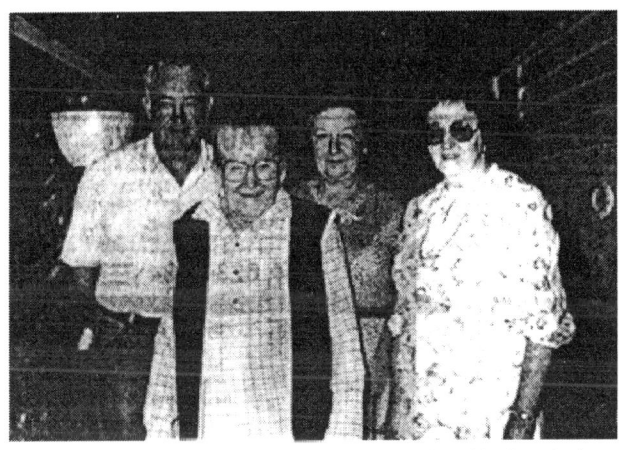

Etta "Granny" Nichols—Last of the Old-Timey Midwives

The Mom claiming the most children was surprised by an early birthday celebration at her home near Blue Mill Road in Del Rio Sunday afternoon. Etta Nichols will turn 90 May 19th and was surrounded by her children on Mother's Day. The midwife likes to think of the over-2000 children she's delivered as some of her own. Her children with her are from left Jack of Del Rio, Belle Smith of Del Rio and June Gilliland of Morristown. (photo by David Popiel)

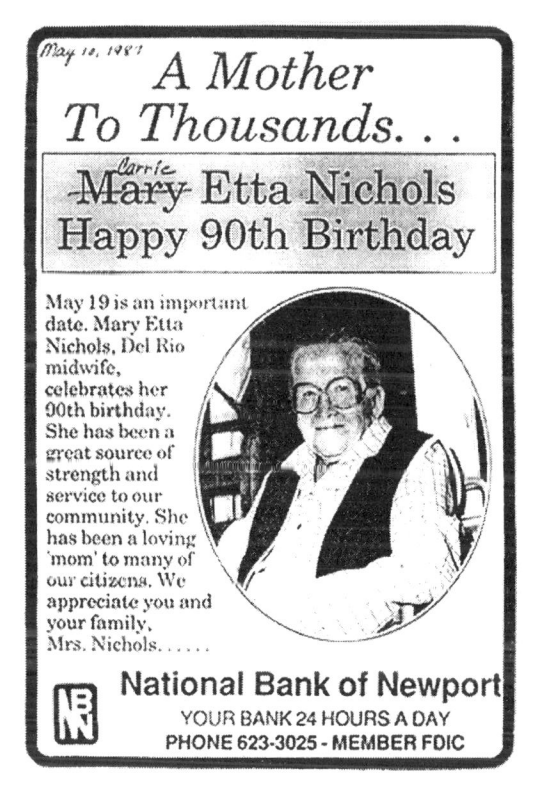

May 10, 1987

A Mother To Thousands...

~~Mary~~ Carrie Etta Nichols
Happy 90th Birthday

May 19 is an important date. Mary Etta Nichols, Del Rio midwife, celebrates her 90th birthday. She has been a great source of strength and service to our community. She has been a loving 'mom' to many of our citizens. We appreciate you and your family, Mrs. Nichols......

National Bank of Newport
YOUR BANK 24 HOURS A DAY
PHONE 623-3025 - MEMBER FDIC

News article and photos courtesy of The Newport Plain Talk.

In June, 1987, Etta received the Humanitarian Award from Douglas-Cherokee, which covered a six-county jurisdiction: Cocke, Grainger, Hamblen, Jefferson, Monroe, and Sevier Counties.

Etta could not attend the award ceremony, so Charles Lewis Moore, Cocke County Executive, and Douglas-Cherokee Board Chairman, Lynn Rouse took the award to her at her home. Also, Wal-Mart placed a large ad in The Newport Plain Talk saluting Etta.

Etta "Granny" Nichols—Last of the Old-Timey Midwives

Agency to honor Del Rio midwife

By Nancy Oberst
City Editor

Her hands have been the first to touch hundreds of babies at the "birthing room" in her immaculate, small home, and hands will be clapping in her honor on Friday night.

Etta Nichols, the Del Rio midwife, has been selected as the recipient of the 1987 Douglas Cherokee Economic Authority Humanitarian Award.

But she will not be able to attend the annual meeting of the Douglas-Cherokee Economic Authority Board of Directors in Morristown on Friday, when her selection will be formally announced.

Jane Joyce, director of the authority's neighborhood centers, said the executive director, Ray McElhaney, will present the award to the midwife "at her convenience" at her home off Ground Squirrel Road.

Mrs. Nichols was selected because "she is the person who best exemplifies the humanitarian qualities; she is a compassionate, caring individual," Joyce said.

The Del Rio woman celebrated her ninetieth birthday on May 19, but she has not retired from being a midwife. She has been practicing midwifery since her 30s. She learned the art from her father, who was a country doctor. She has helped with the births of about 2,000 people, including about 20 sets of twins.

Her midwifery skills have never been used as a moneymaker; she's only charged about $15 for many years. A mother herself, she had four children, one of whom is deceased. She is the grandmother of 13, the great-grandmother of 28, and the great-great-grandmother of two.

Her husband, James Harrison Nichols, suffered a stroke in 1983 and died at home, three years before his wife became internationally known through a National Geographic article about Tennessee.

The humanitarian award to be presented to Mrs. Nichols is presented to someone within the six-county jurisdiction of Douglas-Cherokee: Cocke, Grainger, Hamblen, Jefferson, Monroe, and Sevier counties.

Douglas-Cherokee is an "umbrella agency," which supervises several service organizations, such as Headstart, neighborhood centers, adolescent health programs, an adult literacy program, displaced homemakers, and a senior nutrition program.

The economic authority's board of directors' is made up of 32 representatives -public and private-from the six counties; those from Cocke County are County Executive Charles Lewis Moore, Newport Mayor Jeanne Wilson, Newport Alderman Harold Allen, Lucy Russell, Sam Boger, and alternates Newport Recorder Jack Shepherd and Betty Williams.

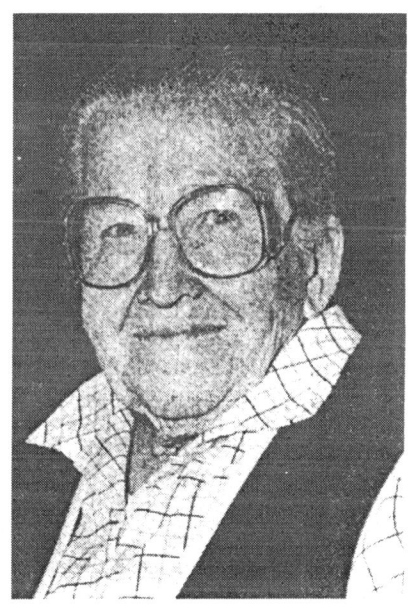

Midwife Etta Nichols

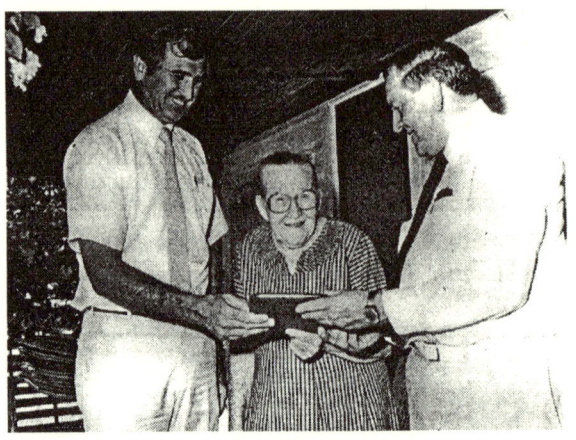

Etta Nichols, the Del Rio midwife, was chosen for the 1987 Douglas-Cherokee Economic Authority Humanitarian Award. She was presented with the award at her home by Cocke County Executive Charles Lewis Moore, left, and Douglas-Cherokee Board Chairman Lynn Rouse. (photo by Nancy Oberst—June 24, 1987)

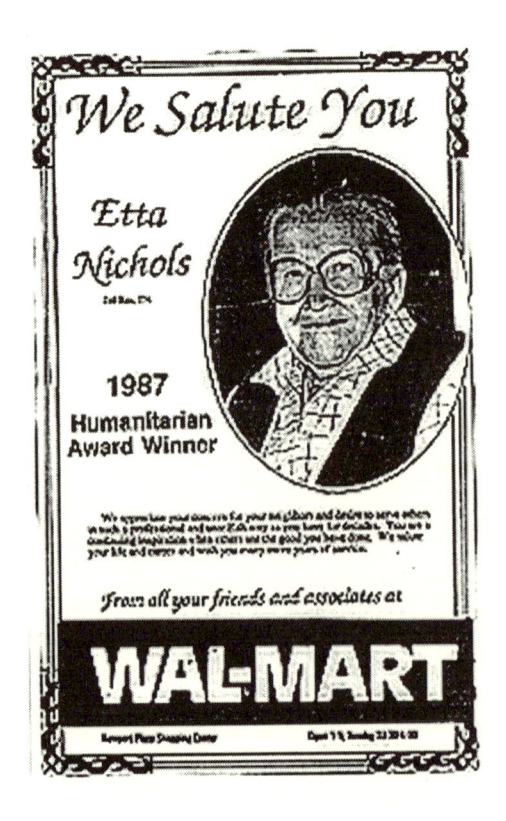

Etta "Granny" Nichols—Last of the Old-Timey Midwives

Humanitarian award winner will continue aiding mothers

By Nancy Oberst
City Editor

Nobody could find Dr. John L. Grigsby when the Moore baby was ready to put in an appearance.

Babies don't wait for doctors, so the next best thing went to Edith Moore's side to wait for the baby, Dr. Grigsby's daughter, Etta Nichols. That baby boy was the first the midwife delivered. She distinctly remembers the birth, but not the boy's name nor how to spell his father's name, which sounded like "Beulo."

A little more than 50 years later, another Moore went to Mrs. Nichols' side Monday afternoon to help present the 1987 Douglas-Cherokee Economic Authority Humanitarian Award. Cocke County Executive Charles Lewis Moore had nominated Mrs. Nichols for the honor.

Douglas-Cherokee's official dinner to honor Mrs. Nichols was on June 12 in Morristown.

She didn't attend the dinner for the award's tenth year, not because she was ill or too feeble to attend. She goes to church every Sunday at Round Mountain Baptist Church and she's still delivering babies. She just saw no point in being honored for something she's done.

"Everything I've done, I haven't done to get my name in anything," she said.

However, "I feel good about it," she said, referring to the recognition she has received for her work. But she just does not understand why she has received such recognition for simply delivering babies.

She has delivered about 2,000 babies, either in the mothers' homes or in the 'birthing room" at her Del Rio home. Many doctors have delivered more than she has, but not after sitting by the mother's side for hours on end and charging no more than $15.

This is why she received her most recent recognition: I feel that no one has done any more for the welfare of Cocke County than Mrs. Nichols, Granny Nichols," said Charles Lewis Moore.

Undaunted by Mrs. Nichols not going to Morristown to pick up her plaque, the plaque-presenters went to the mountains. They got lost, which is understandable, because Mrs. Nichols lives way up in Del Rio, off Ground Squirrel Road right past where State Highway 107 becomes a gravel path as it heads to North Carolina.

But they found her, and County Executive Moore and Douglas-Cherokee Board of Directors Chair-man Lynn Rouse, of Morristown, gave her a plaque for her gift of herself to the community on her front porch. Ray McElhaney, the director of Douglas-Cherokee, and Judi Chobanian, director of the local neighborhood center, also attended the presentation on the mountain woman's porch, along with Mrs. Nichols' favorite dog, a black Chihuahua named Spider.

Mrs. Nichols, who is often called "Granny Nichols," told the group, "you find anybody who's going to have triplets and send them my way."

She doesn't intend to retire from midwifery "until my toes are sticking up," she said. She has delivered 22 or 23 sets of twins, but "I hope to live to deliver triplets."

She has a delivery that "will be any day," and other deliveries "scattered up to November."

In years past, "I've delivered them with only about 10 months apart. A woman keep that up much, she'll lose all her strength," she said, adding she thinks babies ought to be at least two years apart.

She's assisted mothers who were as young as 13 and as old as about 47 or 48. "Some of them are girls and some of them be the last ones," she said.

Of the girls who became mothers in her birthing room, she hasn't counseled them to wait a while, because she didn't think it would do any good, she said. "They wouldn't listen no way."

During the labor pains and the birth, teenage girls have screamed they wouldn't ever have another baby. "I've said I've heard the wind blow, too. They say they won't have no more, but they will."

Just how old was she when she had her first baby? Seventy-one years ago, she was 19 years old when she married Harrison Nichols on October 15. With a glint in her eyes, she said, "I was married nine months and two weeks when my first one was born."

Then and now, she doesn't believe in anything for the pain in giving birth. She has relented in recent years, though, and does have aspirin and Tylenol on hand for mothers.

When she was having her four babies, "the harder my pains, the harder I'd have to bear it. I gritted my teeth. It takes pain to have a baby."

News article and photos courtesy of The Newport Plain Talk.

223

In July 1987, Etta delivered her 23rd set of twins at the age of 90. Gary and Linda Stuart were only expecting one baby, but were blessed with two, born on different days. Alicia Nicole was born at 11:40 P.M. on a Monday night, and Gary Christopher was born at 1:45 A.M. on Tuesday morning.

<u>Newport Plain Talk</u> staff writer Linda McGlasson interviewed the happy parents at Etta's home and wrote the following article:

At 90 Del Rio midwife takes twins in stride

By Linda McGlasson
Staff Writer

A twin treat for a pair of patient parents arrived Monday night and Tuesday morning at Etta Nichol's home in Del Rio.

Gary and Alicia Stuart surprised their parents, who were expecting just one baby but had two, with different birthdays.

Ninety-year-old midwife Etta Nichols delivered her twenty-third set of twins in her career as one of the best-known midwives in the United States.

Until Gary and Linda Stuart arrived at Etta Nichols' home early Monday morning, they didn't have any idea Linda would deliver twins. When they arrived, Etta promptly told Linda she would probably have two, although she was carrying them differently.

Alicia Nicole was born at 11:40 P.M. on Monday, and less than three hours later, her brother, Gary Christopher, joined her at 1:45 A.M. on Tuesday.

After Alicia was born, "and I looked down and I still had this big hump on my stomach, I knew I was going to have another one," Linda said.

Although she stopped working at Regency Health Care Center in April, expecting to have her baby in late May, Linda kept waiting, and waiting. Her husband works at Eastern Plating.

"There at the last I started suspecting I was carrying two, because I was waiting a long time, and also I gained a lot of weight," she said. During her pregnancy, she gained 35 pounds, she said.

The Stuarts are already gearing up to take care of their two new arrivals who were greeted with a bit of apprehension by their two-year-old sister, Julie.

The tired, but elated mother got up Tuesday afternoon for the first time since delivery, to hold her new babies.

Julie will adjust to them; she likes babies," said Linda, as she held her son, Gary.

An extra baby bed has been arranged for the extra arrival, and some extra clothes and diapers are also being taken care of by family members.

Husband and new father Gary was also excited about his twins. When asked about future additions to his family, Stuart said, "This is it." His wife agreed.

Grandparents on both sides of their family have been notified, and "are real happy." Grandparents of the twins are Nelson Hux, of Parrotsville, and the late Jettie Hux; and Arlie Stuart, of Newport, and Evelyn Stuart, of White Pine.

Linda, who works as a resident care assistant at Regency, decided to come to Etta Nichols' house to have her second delivery. Her daughter, Julie, was also a Etta Nichols baby.

"It feels more like home here. In a hospital, it is so foreign and sterile. I feel comfortable here," Linda said. And unlike hospitals, Nichols allows mothers to get up when they feel strong enough, she said. The Stuarts arrived home with their new babies on Tuesday evening.

The twenty-third set of twins were easy to deliver for Etta Nichols, who recently turned 90. "There might have been more twins, but I didn't start counting until several years ago," she said.

She also noted both babies were as large as normal single deliveries. Alicia weighed six pounds and twelve ounces; and Gary weighed seven pounds and eight ounces.

Etta Nichols said she hopes to deliver several more sets of twins, "and if you see anyone who is going to have triplets, send them up here. I've never delivered a trio before," she said, her eyes twinkling, "I wouldn't charge them anything."

Sharon Smith-Ledford

July 24, 1987

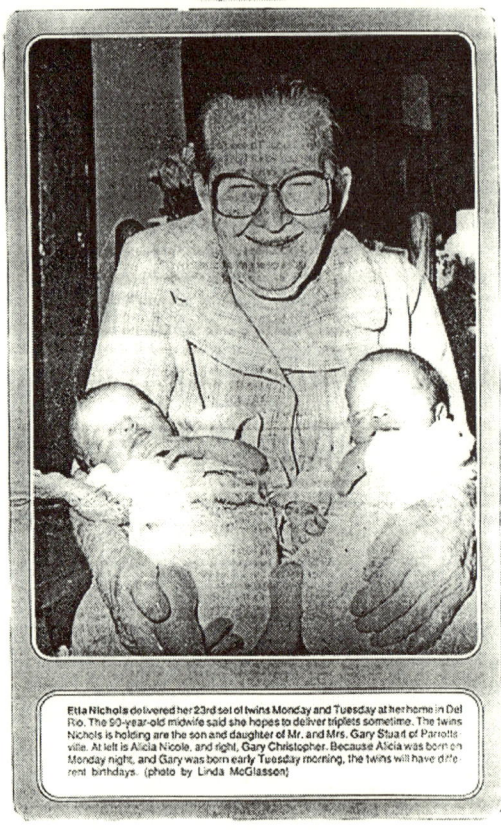

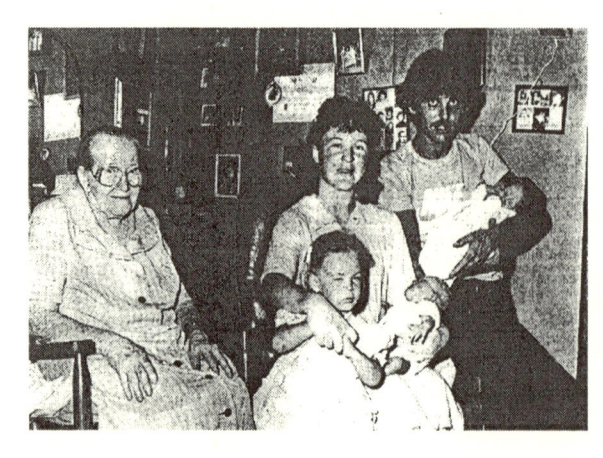

Etta Nichols delivered her 23rd set of twins Monday and Tuesday at her home in Del Rio. The 90-year-old midwife said she hopes to deliver triplets sometime. The twins Nichols is holding are the son and daughter of Mr. and Mrs. Gary Stuart of Parrottsville. At left is Alicia Nicole, and right, Gary Christopher. Because Alicia was born on Monday night, and Gary was born early Tuesday morning, the twins will have different birthdays. (photo by Linda McGlasson)

The Gary Stuart family got double their expectations this week, when Linda Stuart had twins. The Stuart twins make Etta Nichols' record jump to 23 sets of twins delivered in her career as a Del Rio midwife. From left are Nichols, and the Stuart family, Julie Linda's daughter; Linda and Alicia Nichole; and Gary Stuart and his new som Gary Christopher. (photo by Linda McGlasson)

News article and photos courtesy of The Newport Plain Talk.

226

Etta had been having trouble with some of the neighboring dogs coming around trying to kill her goats. One of the dogs bit one of the smaller goats on the back leg, and Etta had to call the vet to nurse it back to health. The goat's leg healed, but it never did walk right again. One afternoon when Etta was going to do her evening milking she discovered one of the baby goats lying lifeless in the field. It had been brutally attacked by the dogs. Etta carried it back to her house and sat up with it all night tending to its wounds and petting it. The next morning the baby goat died. Etta was crushed. She decided then and there she needed to find another home for her goats before the dogs killed any more of them. She called up some friends and told them they could have every one of them if they would come and get them. Her friends agreed to take the goats. Etta's children had been trying to get her to give the goats away ever since one of them butted her and knocked her down, but Etta would not; she loved her goats. But now she was willing to give them up in order to save their lives. Etta's children hated to see their mother saddened so deeply by giving up her goats, but they were also relieved to not have to worry about the goats knocking her down again.

Another year had passed. Etta celebrated her 91st birthday on May 19, 1988. She still lived in her home with Hassa Lee Raines as her live-in companion, and she was still getting around like a 60-year-old. Nancy L. O'Neil, who interviewed Etta on her birthday for The Newport Plain Talk, asked, "What keeps you so young?"

"Hard work. If you sit down and give up you'll become wrinkled and old," Etta laughed.

Sharon Smith-Ledford

FROM THE RECORD—

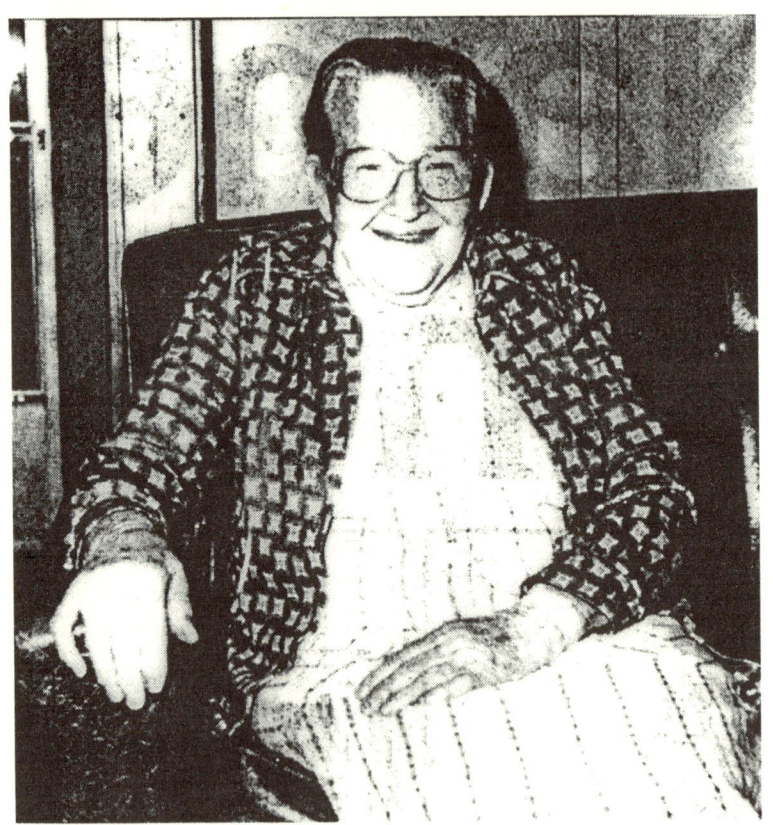

Etta Nichols-Del Rio midwife—She's celebrating 91st

Nancy L. O'Neil
Lifestyle Editor

"Sunrise, sunset, swiftly fly the days..."

Mrs. Etta Nichols, called "Granny" by just about everybody in Del Rio, has seen a lot of them. She celebrated her 91st birthday May 19. Born and reared in Del Rio "across the hill" from where she now lives, she was the oldest daughter of John and Nova Turner Grigsby. Of the seven brothers and sisters three are deceased.

Three of Etta and her husband, Harrison's four children, Belle Smith, Jack Nichols, and June Gilliland are still living. Mrs. Nichols has 13 grandchildren, 22 great-grandchildren, and two great-great-grandchildren.

Visiting with this spry lady with twinkling eyes no one would believe she is 91. Yet, between questions and answers, her telephone rings again and again with well wishers calling to congratulate her. "Come see me," she tells each one. "I'm hungry for the sight of you."

What keeps her so young? "Hard work. If you sit down and give up you'll become wrinkled and old," she laughed. Women have come from near and far requesting her assistance bringing their children into the world. In her career as a mid-wife, she has birthed more than 2,000 babies including 22 sets of twins. "I'd like to birth a set of triplets before I die," she said.

What about retirement? "I'll do that when my toes are sticking up," she laughed.

News article and photos courtesy of The Newport Plain Talk.

Etta "Granny" Nichols—Last of the Old-Timey Midwives

In the year 1989, one week before Etta turned 92 years old, she unknowingly delivered the last child she would help bring into the world. It was a little girl. A woman who was studying midwifery came with the expectant mother and helped with the delivery.

Some months later, Etta developed a blood clot in her side and had to be taken to Cocke County Baptist Hospital. Dr. Williams was her doctor. She remained hospitalized for 12 days. While Etta was in the hospital she had congestive heart failure. Her blood pressure went so low the doctor thought he was going to lose her, but Etta was always a strong-willed, and healthy woman. She had no intentions of leaving just yet. When she was released from the hospital, she stayed with Belle, but she wanted to go back to her own home. One day a woman came to Belle's house, whose children Etta had delivered, to visit Etta. Belle mentioned she was searching for someone to stay with Etta so she could move back to her own house. Hassa Lee had moved into a house trailer on some property beside Etta and would no longer be staying with her. The woman told Belle she would stay with Etta until the day she died. Etta was thrilled; she got to move back home. But three weeks later the woman left, and wasn't planning on coming back. She had left her son to live in her house and care for it, but he had moved out, so she had to move back home.

Knowing how much it meant to Etta, Belle went over and stayed with her mother during the day so Etta could remain in her own home. After Etta went to bed at night, Belle went back to her own home. Margaret Stokley, or her sister, Shirley, stayed with Etta at night most of the time. This arrangement continued for several months, then Etta got another blood clot in her leg. Dr. Williams told Etta she must stay off her feet or she would risk having the blood clot travel up to her heart and kill her. Belle had no choice but to move Etta back in with her where she could care for her properly.

Etta had delivered over 2,000 babies during her career as a midwife, which included 23 sets of twins. The smallest baby she delivered weighed 1 1/2 pounds, and lived. The largest baby weighed 14 pounds...and the mother lived! Etta never lost a baby in birth, though a few were stillborn. Etta took in mothers as young as 13 and as old as 48. During her years of practice Etta lost only one patient. Etta told the woman she needed to go to the hospital, or she would risk dying, but because of the woman's religious beliefs, she would not go. She died giving birth, but the baby survived. Etta was deeply saddened that the woman had not listened to her. Now her baby would grow up never knowing his mother.

Etta had many different types of experiences as a midwife, and had made many new friends in the process. One mother liked Etta so much she named her baby, Carrie Etta. Every expectant mother left Etta's house saying she enjoyed her stay there, but the time had come when she could no longer care for the women. She had always said she would retire "when her toes were sticking straight up," but due to ill health, she was forced to give it up before that day came. It saddened Etta to know she would no longer be able to help bring these brand-new lives into the world. How she loved her babies! The part of her life that had brought her so much joy through the years was now over. The day had come for Etta to retire from being a midwife.

Part VII

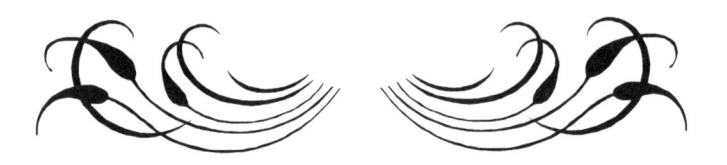

Heaven Awaits

Part VII

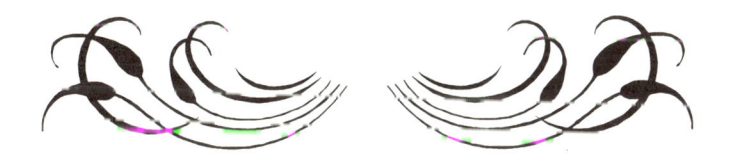

Heaven Awaits

Etta took turns staying with her daughters June and Belle. She was staying with June during the Christmas of 1989. Floyd, Belle, and Sharon all went to June's house in Morristown to celebrate with Etta on Christmas Day. June's children, and grandchildren were all there, too. Everyone sat around in the living room and watched as Etta opened her gifts. She received many nice presents from her family. After all the gifts were opened, Etta walked to the kitchen table with only the help of John holding her hand. She still got around well for a person of 93. It was plain to see Etta had enjoyed her day with her family gathered around her.

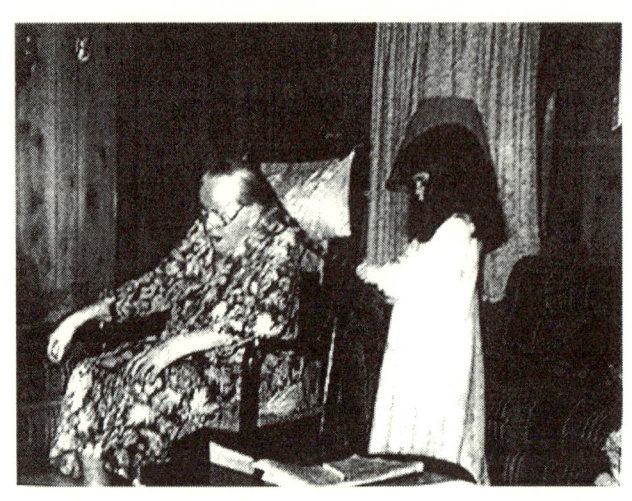

Katie Hayes, Etta's great-granddaughter, braids Etta's hair before going to bed.

That night Johnnie Sue and her daughter, Katie, stayed with John and June. Katie loved braiding Etta's long hair, and Etta seemed to enjoy it, too.

On May 1, 1990, Etta moved back to Belle's house to give June a break. Etta had a walker now which she had to use to get around, but she managed just fine going from room to room by herself. Belle had two full-size beds in her bedroom—Belle slept in one, and Etta in the other. Floyd slept in the back bedroom so his snoring would not disturb them.

Smoky Mountain Home Health had brought Etta a hospital bed before she ever left her home, so Belle had it moved into her bedroom to make it easier to help Etta in and out of the bed by raising or lowering the head of the mattress.

Etta started her day by getting a refreshing sponge bath and getting dressed. Breakfast followed, usually one scrambled egg, toast, and Postum, sometimes oatmeal. After breakfast Etta sat in her lift chair in the living room, which raised up and down to help her get in and out of it, and started piecing on the handmade quilt she worked on every day. At the age of 93 Etta could still see well enough to thread her own needle, although if the needle had a very small eye, she had to get Belle or Venida to thread it for her. Etta sat for hours sewing the quilt pieces together day after day. It seemed to give a purpose for her to go on.

Since all the family knew Etta would not be returning to her home again to live, Belle, who had power of attorney, discussed with Etta the idea of going ahead and selling her house. "Someone needs to be living in it, Mother, so it won't just set there and ruin," Belle told her.

Etta agreed it would be for the best. She told Belle to go ahead and give her furniture and belongings to the family members she specified so the house would be empty in case someone wanted to buy it.

The next day at Belle's house, Belle asked Venida and Sharon what they wanted from the items left over after June, Jack, and she had taken what Etta had told them to take.

"I told Mamaw I don't know how many times that I wanted that wooden rocking chair if she ever decided to get rid of it, but she gave it to one of the other grandchildren, so it I could have one of her homemade quilts, it would make me happy," said Sharon.

"Honey, I'm sorry. She gave every one of her quilts away to some woman that came up there to have a baby. The woman had some little kids, and they told Mother they wished they could stay nice and warm like they did at her house. They said they couldn't stay warm at their house, so Mother gave them every quilt she had," Belle answered.

"What! Didn't she think any of her children, or grandchildren, might want one of her quilts for a keepsake someday? Well, that's Mamaw for you. She'd give the shirt off her back if it would help someone. I guess I shouldn't be selfish. Tell her I want her to make me a quilt when she finishes the one she's working on now."

"Is there anything else you'd like, since you didn't get the rocker, or a quilt? She has some antique dishes and stuff in the kitchen, and I know you said you like antiques," Belle offered.

"Yeah, that'll be fine. I just want something of hers to remember her by," Sharon answered.

It seemed kind of strange, and sad, to everyone in the family to be passing out Etta's belongings before she had died, but with the house going up for sale there was no place to store them; it was the only solution.

Several months passed before Etta's house was sold. Arthell Moore, a resident of Del Rio, bought it. Belle could tell it disturbed her mother when she told her the news. Etta had almost 60 years of happy memories living in that house. It was hard for Etta to say good-bye, knowing this time it was final.

During Etta's stay with Belle this time, June developed shingles and was not well enough to care for her mother any more. Also, June's bedroom doors were too narrow to allow a hospital bed to enter through them, and Etta had to have a hospital bed in order to get in and out of it. So it was decided between June and Belle that their mother would have to remain with Belle, probably for the rest of her life. June and other family members agreed to come and sit with Etta whenever Belle needed to run errands. Nellie Stokley Haney, the little girl Etta had helped cure from a case of rheumatic fever when she was 11 years old, also came to sit with Etta when Belle needed someone. Nellie thought the world of Etta, and was always willing to do anything she could to help with her. One day Nellie and her mother-in-law, Hattie Haney, came to visit with Etta. She wanted a picture of herself with this woman who had done so much for her family, and the community, so Belle got out her camera and took a picture of the three ladies together. Nellie stands on the right, and Mrs. Haney stands on the left.

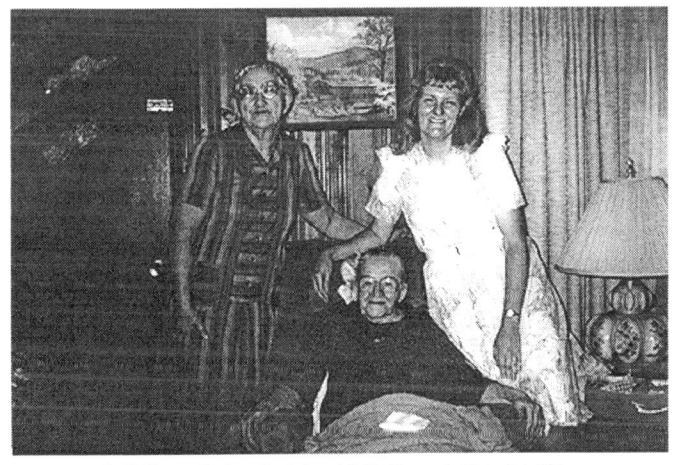

Hattie Haney stands on the left, and Nellie Haney stands on the right

Belle's husband, Floyd, had been diagnosed with lung cancer after having tests run at Saint Mary's Hospital in Knoxville during the spring of 1991. The cancer was caused from a job Floyd worked on in his earlier years where he was exposed to asbestos. Belle and the rest of the family were devastated by the news. Floyd received many visits from old friends and family members once the news spread about his illness.

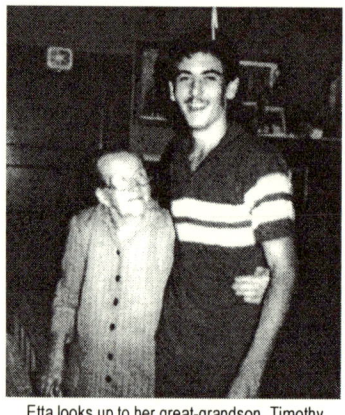

On October 17, 1991, Etta lost one of her great-grandsons. Valerie's only son, Timothy Thornton, was killed in an auto crash at the age of 23. Valerie had five girls who were born before Timothy— Vicki, Kim, Lisa, Sherry, and Karen. He was the youngest child. The funeral was held at Manes Funeral Home in Newport. Timothy was laid to rest in the Chestnut Hill Methodist Cemetery.

Etta looks up to her great-grandson, Timothy Thornton, Age 18 in this photo

When Winter arrived in 1991, Floyd's illness had progressed to the point where he could no longer get around without becoming exhausted. Belle ordered another hospital bed and had it placed in the dinning room so Floyd could stay in bed and rest, but still be close to her while she worked in the kitchen.

Christmas Eve of 1991 arrived. All of Belle's family, children and grandchildren, came to Floyd and Belle's on Christmas Eve to exchange gifts and eat Christmas dinner so they could spend Christmas Day at their own homes. This Christmas was not like the ones before, though. There was a sadness in the air because the family knew this would be the last Christmas they would get to spend with their loved one, Floyd, yet everyone tried to be strong and cheerful for his sake.

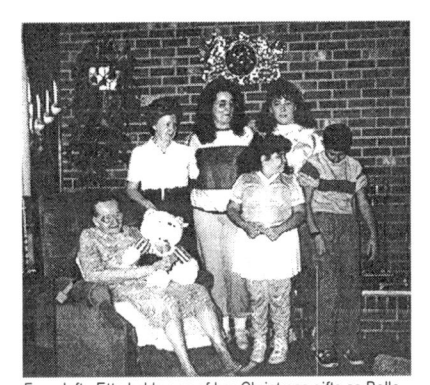

Etta "Granny" Nichols—Last of the Old-Timey Midwives

From left: Etta holds one of her Christmas gifts as Belle, Venida, and her children, Felicia, Mark, and Amanda Guillot pose beside Etta for a Christmas snapshot.

Etta sat in her lift chair and opened her gifts. One of her presents was a beautiful, snuggly, white teddy bear. Etta held it close to her and would not even let it go while she had her Christmas snap shots made with the family.

Floyd had given Venida some money to buy her children some Christmas gifts from him. One of the presents Venida chose for her youngest daughter, Amanda, was a little white cockapoo puppy. Amanda was so excited, she loved it as soon as she saw it. Amanda chose to name her first puppy Sarah. Amanda took Sarah to Etta and let Etta hold her. Etta seemed thrilled as she wrapped the puppy in the blanket she had covering her legs. She stroked the puppy affectionately and talked baby talk to it for hours. When Amanda went back to get her dog from Etta she ran into a bit of a problem. Etta did not want to let the puppy go; she apparently misunderstood and thought the puppy belonged to her. Finally, Venida intervened and explained to her grandmother that the puppy belonged to

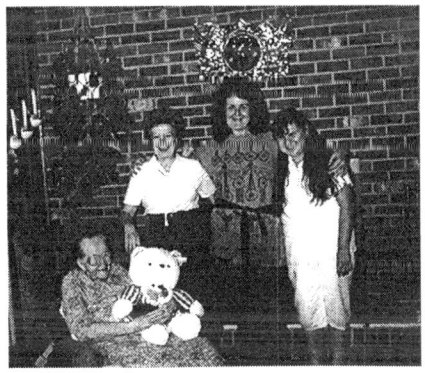

Belle, Sharon Kay, and her daughter, Tiffany Alise, also pose for a four-generation Christmas snapshot.

Amanda. Etta frowned at Amanda strongly as Venida picked up the puppy from Etta's lap and handed it to Amanda. It hurt Venida knowing she had to take the dog from Etta. Etta had always been a strong animal lover, and showed real happiness as she stroked the puppy. Venida handed the teddy bear that Etta had received as a gift back to her, and it seemed to calm her as she wrapped her arm around it.

Belle had always been a very good cook, and at Christmas time there was always a feast fit for a king sitting on her dinning room table. Each of her children would bring a dish, or some drinks, also. There was turkey, turkey dressing, gravy, ham, green beans from the garden, creamed-style corn from the garden, slaw, potato salad, yams, whipped potatoes, cranberry sauce, rolls, and cornbread. And there were usually six or seven different types of desserts to choose from. After the meal was over, and the kitchen was cleaned, everyone retired to the living room. Some fell asleep in their chairs for a short afternoon nap, while others looked at old photographs, or read a magazine. It was a time everyone cherished, being together with the entire family and showing their love for one another on a very special day.

Lynda and her family had been living in Newark, Ohio, for the past seven or eight years, but had come home to spend Christmas with the family. Lynda was reluctant to leave to return to Ohio because her father's health seemed to be deteriorating rapidly. She called her daughter Renina, who also lived in Ohio, and told her she needed to make plans to come to Del Rio because she felt her father did not have many more days to live.

On Monday, December 31, 1991, all the family was at Belle's house. It had been decided that it was time to take Floyd to Cocke County Baptist Hospital in Newport to spend the remainder of the days he had left. They could give him medicine to help reduce his pain. An ambulance was called to come pick Floyd up at his house. Everyone knew that when Floyd left he would never be coming back. The family stood in the dining room weeping as they kissed him and shared some final precious moments together. Etta sat in her lift chair in the living room watching as everyone sobbed in the next room. Although she did not realize why everyone was crying, she began to cry, too. She knew something terribly sad was going on, and she cried for the pain her family was feeling.

Floyd spent four days in the hospital, with different family members taking turns staying with him. Lynda was staying with her dad on Thursday night when he suddenly had a seizure. She called for the nurses immediately. The rest of the family was called to come to the hospital—it was time to say one final good-bye. Floyd took his last breath at 12:10 A.M. on January 3, 1992. All the family was in the room with him during his passing. Floyd's funeral was held at 8 P.M. on Saturday night at Brown's Funeral Home in Newport, with Rev. Tois Seay officiating. At 10:30 A.M. Sunday morning, Floyd Jay Smith was laid to rest in the Clark Cemetery on Midway Road in Del Rio.

More bad news came for Etta upon hearing about the death of her sister, Willie, who died on April 18, 1992. Etta was unable to attend the services, but her thoughts and her heart was with her dear, departed sister. Emily

Willie Grigsby was laid to rest in the Jonestown Cemetery in a plot beside where Etta would someday rest beside her husband, Harrison.

On May 19, 1992, Etta celebrated her 95th birthday. She had already lived much longer than the family expected her to. Belle continued caring for her mother in her home, although Belle was tired and weak, she was not about to let her mother be taken to a nursing home to spend her last years. She had been too good of a person to be neglected by her family now.

In September 1992, Etta received an injury to her hip and was no longer able to walk. From then on she was confined to her bed.

On October 25, 1992, Etta's brother, Lurlie, passed away. When Belle told Etta the painful news, she seemed to forget all about it in just a few minutes. Her mind was no longer able to remember, or concentrate on certain things for very long periods of time any more. Lurlie Grigsby was buried at the Mulberry Cemetery.

All of Etta's younger siblings, except Alverta and Furman, had passed on before her.

Venida and her husband, David, had moved their family into Belle's house so she could help her mother tend to Etta. One evening one of Belle's cousins, Dorothy Martin, and her husband, Albert, from Hayesville, North Carolina, came by to visit before going back home. Venida and David were in the kitchen eating supper, while Belle entertained her visitors in the living room. Etta realized there was company in the house, and in her mind she prepared everyone a large meal and hollered out, "Supper, Supper!"

Etta "Granny" Nichols—Last of the Old-Timey Midwives

Venida and David looked at each other in bewilderment as they wondered if they had heard Etta correctly. Again Etta hollered out, "Supper!" only this time she sounded really agitated. Venida and David went in to see what Etta wanted.

"I've cooked supper, but I can't get anybody to come and eat it," Etta said pointing towards the dresser as if it was her stove. "I've got beans, potatoes, cornbread, and all kinds of stuff on the stove over there," Etta continued.

Venida and David walked over to the dresser and pretended to eat the food she had prepared in her mind. "Boy, this sure is good, Mamaw," said David. Venida told her she sure did appreciate the delicious meal she had fixed for them. Venida and David's comments seemed to please Etta. After all, she had not gone to all that trouble to just let it sit there and ruin.

Etta's memory continued to weaken to the point that she sometimes did not even recognize Belle, and she called the pictures of Belle's children on the wall her own babies. Sometimes her mind regressed back to when she was a little girl, and she would ask questions about people she knew as a child. One day she started talking about a neighbor who had come to her house and killed one of her pet chickens to eat. "He walked up and grabbed my chicken and whacked its head off!" Etta said with emotion. "And that night they had chicken 'n dumplin's for supper! Yeah, he just whacked its head off!!" Venida tried not to laugh as her grandmother continued, but some of her stories were so funny it was hard not to.

Etta received many visitors before and after she became bedfast. Albert and Dorothy Martin, Belle's first cousin on her daddy's side; Willie's daughter, Ruth, and her family; Hobert and Lucy Nichols, related on Harrison's side, and Rev. Robert Ashley, and his wife, Shirley, just to name a few. Church groups came by with fruit baskets and sang songs to Etta, and, of course, all of her children and grandchildren visited as often as possible.

Sometimes Etta took "hyper spells." She would talk and talk. When she did this she wanted someone in the room with her constantly to talk to. One such spell lasted for three days and two nights, keeping Belle awake. During her hyper spells Etta told some of the funniest stories, things Belle had never heard her talk about before. Belle decided the next time her mother had a hyper spell she was going to call her brother, Jack, who lived in the valley behind her house. Belle wanted Jack to hear some of their mother's stories. So, a few weeks later Etta began to have another hyper spell. Belle called Jack, and he came up and stayed several hours by Etta's bedside. Etta had been worrying about her chickens all day and was trying to get someone to take her to her house so she could feed them and put them up for the night. David had promised her he would look after her chickens, but when Jack walked in her room, she started on him about her chickens, too. Although Etta no longer owned chickens, or her house, the family went along with her. Jack promised to go feed her chickens and put them up for the night. That seemed to satisfy Etta. She began talking about a house she had lived in before they moved into the one on Ground Squirrel. Her mind was hardly ever on the present anymore, but had regressed to living in the past.

Christmas of 1993 came. Belle's family gathered at her house on Christmas Eve as always. It was apparent everyone was saddened because Floyd wasn't there to share this special time with the family, but everyone tried to keep their spirits up for the children's sake. Etta received many nice gifts. One gift from Belle was a baby doll that was the next thing to being real. Etta held the doll close to her in her bed, and wrapped it up in her blanket. She loved it. When Belle went back into the room to check on Etta she noticed her mother was just working away, rubbing the doll's legs and arms, and trying to wrap the covers around it.

"This baby is so cold, and no matter what I do I can't get it warm," Etta told Belle in a worried tone. Belle got another small blanket and wrapped the doll up in it. "It'll be warm now, Mother. Just let it lay here beside you."

Etta thought the doll was a real baby, which only showed that even in her old age, she still adored babies, and was still kind and very concerned about their well-being.

Some nurses from Smoky Mountain Home Health had started coming to help with Etta two or three times a week. They bathed her, took her blood pressure, changed her sheets, and did anything else Etta needed them to do. One day as one of the nurses was bathing Etta, she looked up at her and said, "Well, I reckon women have quit havin' babies. I haven't had any patients in I don't know when."

"Oh no, they're still having babies, Mrs. Nichols. They have to go to the hospital now to have them," the nurse answered. She got tickled because Etta thought if women weren't coming to her, they must not be having babies anymore.

Bad news hit the family again on March 11, 1994. June's husband, John, had a massive heart attack and died in his living room. John was well liked by the entire family and would definitely be missed. Funeral services were held at Calvary Baptist Church in Morristown, and John was laid to rest in the Jarnigan Cemetery, also in Morristown.

Having only three grandsons, Etta held a special place in her heart for them. Darrell, Emily's son, had always been very close to his grandmother. He held his marriage ceremony to his wife, Janice, at Etta's house on Christmas Day, 1976. They were married by Esq. Jack Barrett. Darrell loved farm animals just like Etta did. He helped Etta all he could after Harrison died. When Etta became bedfast, Darrell could not bring himself to visit her. He said he just could not stand to see her that way; he wanted to remember her as she was before. It probably did not matter anyway, because Etta hardly ever recognized family members anymore.

On July 2, 1994, Darrell had a fatal heart attack while driving to town with his wife, Janice.

The news came as a terrible shock to the entire family. Darrell had only turned 40 on May 20th, and now he was gone. The funeral was held at Westside Funeral Home in Morristown. Charles Richard Darrell Jones was laid to rest in the Jarnigan Cemetery.

No one told Etta about the death of her grandson. If she had remembered who he was, it would only have upset her deeply. The family saw no need to put her through the pain.

In early September 1994, Etta received a surprise visitor. Belle, Venida, and James Taylor helped Alverta from the motor home her son drove from Florida to come visit Etta. When Alverta entered Etta's room, Etta's face lit up with excitement as she exclaimed, "Well, here comes Alvertie!"

Alverta sat down on Belle's bed which was beside Etta's bed. The two ladies reminisced about things of the past. It seemed to the other family members that seeing Alverta had brought back Etta's entire memory of the past, until Etta looked over at Alverta and asked, "How's Poppy doin'?"

Alverta looked over at Venida sitting beside her, with an expression of bewilderment. Alverta pointed her finger toward heaven with a sad expression on her face to indicate to Etta that their father had died.

"You mean Poppy's dead?" Etta asked in a puzzled tone.

Alverta shook her head yes.

"Well, nobody told me!" Etta said in an almost aggravated tone.

"Poppy sure was a good one," Alverta said.

After visiting with one another for awhile longer it was time for Alverta and Etta to say their good-byes. Alverta seemed to know this would be the last time she would see Etta in this lifetime. Tears filled Alverta's eyes as she leaned over Etta's bed and said, "Now, I'll pray for you, and you pray for me."

Etta was choked up as she answered, "I will."

Etta's family was afraid Etta would be upset after Alverta left, but she seemed to forget all about her visit. God had apparently allowed Etta's memory to return long enough for these two sisters to have one last precious visit together.

On November 18, 1994, Belle was awakened around 3 A.M. by her mother. "She was singing the prettiest song, and she spoke her words so clearly. It was almost as if she knew something was about to happen," Belle told her children the following day.

Later that day Etta had a stroke, leaving her throat paralyzed. Pat Hurley, the nurse from Smoky Mountain Home Health, said Etta would probably do well to live another week. She was no longer able to eat or drink because the stroke prevented her from swallowing. Pat had been caring for Etta for several months, and she had become very fond of her. Pat had accepted another job so when she left Etta this time she knew she would not be seeing her again, and she knew Etta did not have many more days to live. As Pat left the house tears streamed down her cheeks. She would certainly miss this sweet little old lady.

The following week was a true test of faith for Etta's family. Exactly one week later, on Friday, November 25, 1994, Etta lay in her twin-size hospital bed between clean white sheets and a pale blue blanket which covered her frail, withered body. Her waist-length brown- and- gray hair lay plaited in one large strand by her side. It shimmered in the illuminating sunlight which beamed through the windows opposite her bed. Snow-white strands framed her face, creating a softness around her beautiful blue eyes, which one only earns through graciousness. A white antique chest stood in the room toward the foot of Etta's bed; a matching dresser sat along the right wall at the foot of Belle's bed. A beautiful blue water pitcher and basin rested on top of the chest while the dresser held family pictures and other odds and ends. On Belle's headboard two small reading lamps, and a stuffed koala bear from Australia which Floyd Ray had sent to his mother during his tour in Vietnam. The Holy Bible lay alongside the Sunday school lesson for the following Sunday's church service, which Belle studied while she rested in her bed each night.

Etta seemed quite content to have never been out of the bed for over two years, but she never was one to complain about anything. She accepted life the way God sent it to her, and she made the most of it.

June had been staying with Belle for a few days so she could help Belle with their mother, and to be close to Etta during the time she had left.

On this day, Belle decided she needed to go to Newport to get some medicine for her mother, and to pick up some items at the grocery store. She and her grandson, Darren Burgin, left the house around 10 A.M. They had not been gone long when Venida went to check on her grandmother. Venida noticed Etta's hands were turning blue. She had been told by the nurse, who had been there only a couple of hours earlier, that this was one of the signs to look for to know that death was near. Venida went into the kitchen to call her Uncle Jack, who lived in the peaceful, isolated hollow directly behind Belle's house. Venida informed him, "I think it's time." She waited for

Jack to arrive before telling her Aunt June, who was in the kitchen washing dishes. Jack was there in a matter of minutes. Venida also called her sister, Lynda Burgin, and Lynda's husband, Edd, to come to the house. They also lived close by.

Felicia, Venida's daughter, stood on the right side of her great-grandmother's bed holding her frail, wrinkled hand in hers. Venida, Lynda, and Edd stood at the foot of the bed, while June and Jack stood on the left side of the bed; all waiting for the inevitable. June bent over the cold, silver bedside rails which stretched along the side of the bed, and kissed her mother on the forehead "I love you, Mother," were the last words June said to her.

Etta opened her eyes wide as she looked up at her daughter and her only son standing over her.

"I think she knows you," Felicia said to June.

"No, Honey. She don't know," responded Jack.

Etta closed her eyes and released her last breath at the age of 97.

"I'll bet angels are in this room right now," proclaimed Venida.

It was 10:45 A.M. when Sharon received the shattering news while working at her job in Morristown.

"Sharon, Mamaw just died," came Venida's quavering voice over the phone. Venida gave Sharon the details that had just unfolded. Sharon's eyes filled with tears as she listened. No one could have loved their grandmother more than she did.

Belle and Darren returned home about 30 minutes after Etta's passing. Edd met Belle outside as she approached the front door. "She's gone." Edd said sympathetically.

Belle's eyes opened widely in astonishment. "Oh, she is?" asked Belle in a shocked tone. (It was later discussed among the family members how God must have intended for Belle to be gone when her mother passed away, for she had not left her side for weeks until this very morning at this very hour. He must have known she would not have been able to handle watching her mother take her last breath.)

Belle entered the bedroom she had shared with her mother for the past two years. There she released the tears she had been desperately trying to hold back as she said her final good-bye to her beloved mother.

Etta's funeral was held at Brown's Funeral Home in Newport. The number of people who came to pay their last respects was tremendous. Margaret Carrie Etta Nichols was laid to rest in the Jonestown Cemetery in Del Rio on November 28, at 10 A.M. beside her husband, Harrison Nichols.

At last, Etta was freed from her tired, worn-out body. Her spirit was now free to soar with the angels in Heaven, where she belonged.

• • • • • •

This was the life Etta viewed as she stood in the presence of God. When it came to an end, He held out his arm toward the gates of heaven and said, "Well done, My child. You may enter."

As Etta started toward the gates of Heaven she heard a faint, familiar voice coming from Earth saying, "Etta was one of a kind. She did so much for the people in our community. She was truly the last of the old-timey midwives."

Midwife of the mountains dies

Etta Nichols delivered more than 2,000 babies at Del Rio

The old mountain saying, "A tall woman casts a long shadow," is an apt description of Etta Nichols, a Del Rio resident and midwife who delivered babies for more than half a century.

Nichols, 97, who was affectionately called "Granny," died Friday at the home of her daughter, Belle Smith, in Del Rio.

Local doctors and nurses believe she was the last of the many untrained "granny" midwives who practiced during the pioneer period of East Tennessee and Western North Carolina.

The granddaughter of a doctor and the daughter of a man who had some medical training, she watched her father deliver babies and decided, as she said in a 1985 interview, "Most of what I know I learned by experience. You learn a lot of things out of books and forget them. But you don't forget what you learn by experience."

Because of obligations at home, she never received formal schooling past the eighth grade.

Although she was not able to fulfill her dream of attaining the training to become a nurse, the knowledge learned from her father by watching him deliver babies, led her to deliver more than 2,000 babies, including 23 sets of twins, in her career.

In the early years, the calls would come and she would go to the mother's home to meet the stork. Later, when she was no longer able to travel the hills and hollows of rural Cocke County, she added a room to her home near Round Mountain Baptist Church and the patients came to her.

The delivery room was a nine foot-square room with two beds, a commode, sink, and two medicine cabinet.

In 1985, a film crew from NBC interviewed Nichols, and the program was aired as part of the *Nightly News with Tom Brokaw*.

Despite the fact that her fame spread, she never charged more than $15 per delivery. She said, "If they can't pay, I don't push them. I don't want none of these babies going hungry."

She delivered her last baby when she was a mere 92.

"It takes pains to have a baby," she said, explaining why she didn't administer painkillers.

"They (the mothers) do better if they're not doped up."

None ever needed a Cesarean section, something she attributed to luck and patience.

Though small in stature, everyone who met "Granny" Nichols came away with an impression of a strong, independent woman with a twinkle in her eyes, and the gift of helping in her hands for those most helpless of all, the newborn.

Mrs. Nichols, the widow of James Harrison Nichols, was a member of Bridgeport Free Will Baptist Church.

She was also preceded in death by her daughter, Emily Jones, two grandchildren, and one great-grandchild.

Survivors include her children, June Gilliland, of Morristown; Jack Nichols and Belle Smith, of Del Rio; 12 grandchildren; 27 great-grandchildren; seven great-great-grandchildren; a sister, Alverta Taylor, of Jacksonville, Florida;

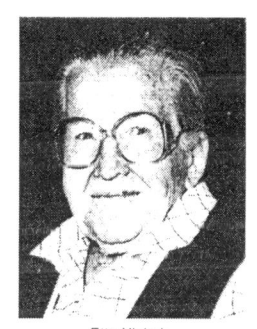

Etta Nichols

and a brother, Furman Grigsby, of Bridgeport.

Services were 8 P.M. Sunday at Brown Funeral Home Chapel with Rev. Robert Ashley and Rev. A. W. Campbell officiating.

Burial was 10 A.M. Monday in the Jones Town Cemetery.

Brown Funeral Home was in charge.

Del Rio
Shirley James

Hello once again! I hope everyone had a wonderful Thanksgiving. Now we know Christmas will soon be here. I hope that with all the planning, shopping and excitement, everyone remembers what Christmas is really all about, Don't forget! It is a very special birthday. Let's keep this in mind while enjoying the festivities.

Well, our community has been saddened by the loss of one of the most special ladies I have ever met—Etta Nichols. She was a midwife who delivered many babies at no worry if there would be any pay or not. She was one of the most kind, generous, giving, Christian persons I have ever been fortunate enough to meet in my lifetime. I remember as a child sitting on a bench behind her very inviting table and eating the most delicious apple pies I ever tasted. I have never forgotten the taste of those pies and probably never will. Our community lost a great asset, but her memory will always linger in our hearts. Granny Nichols' family has our love, sympathy, prayers and thoughts at this bereaved time in their lives. God blessed her with 97 years on this earth, but remember, our loss is Heaven's gain.

Thousands Remember Her Labor

BY ROBERT MOORE
Tribune Staff Writer

DEL RIO—On Thursday, the day before Etta "Granny" Nichols died at the age of 97, her youngest child Belle Smith leaned over Mrs. Nichols' bed and whispered "I love you." Etta managed a smile, looked into her baby's eyes and mouthed the familiar words, "I love you, too, honey."

Mrs. Nichols died on Friday, but because of a 65-year labor of love, thousands are here to remember and honor the memory of a selfless life.

In the early years, the urgent messages came by a rider on horseback, later by telephone—the pains have started and she needs you. Always, in more than 2,000 instances, Granny Nichols was there to deliver the baby.

Although Mrs. Nichols' grandfather was a medical doctor and her father picked up the profession casually, she had only eight years of formal schooling.

The turning point in her life came 64 years ago when a woman went into labor while Mrs. Nichols' father was away on another case. She had watched her father deliver babies and figured there was not much to it.

"I guess it was just in my blood," she said in a 1985 interview, "I always wanted to be a nurse, but I had too much work to do to go to school. My father had a lot of doctor books, but I never had time to read 'em much."

"Most of what I know I learned by experience. You learn a lot of things out of books and forget them. But you don't forget what you learn by experience."

Although Mrs. Nichols' services were invaluable to the people of Cocke County, the services came cheap—fifteen dollars, or less if she felt her patients did not have the money to pay

"Some people can't even pay the $15," she said. "I don't push em'. I don't want none of these babies to going hungry"

Of the 2,000-plus babies Mrs. Nichols' delivered, including at least 23 sets of twins, none of the patients ever required a Caesarian section or heavy anesthesia, something she attributes to good luck and patience.

"The reason these doctors do it so much is they get in too big a hurry," she said. "It takes pains to have a baby; They (the mothers) get along better if they're not all doped up."

About 20 years ago, because of failing health, Mrs. Nichols was forced to suspend housecalls deliveries and started working out of her home in rural Cocke County. She delivered her last baby five years ago at the age of 92.

Mrs. Nichols' daughter, Mrs. Smith, said she has mixed emotions about her mother's death. While mourning is natural, Mrs. Smith says, knowing her mother led a full and rewarding life is a great consolation during times of grief.

"Of course we're glad that she's at rest," Mrs. Smith said. "She had a good life. She just wanted to do things for other people and that's what sticks out in my mind."

Brown's Funeral Home in Newport is in charge of the funeral arrangements.

Mrs. Nichols was a member of Free Will Baptist Church. She was preceded in death by her husband, James Harrison Nichols; daughter, Emily Jones; two grandchildren and one great-grandson.

Survivors include her daughters, June Gilliland of Morristown and Belle Smith of Del Rio; son, Jack Nichols of Del Rio; 12 grandchildren; 27 great-grandchildren; seven great-great grandchildren; sister, Alverta Taylor of Jacksonville, Fla.; and brother, Furman Grigsby of Bridgeport.

Funeral services will be held at 8 P.M. today at the Brown's Funeral Home Chapel with the Revs. Robert Ashley and A. W. Campbell officiating. The family will receive friends from 6-8 P.M. prior to the services.

Burial will be at 10 A.M. Monday in the Jonestown Cemetery.

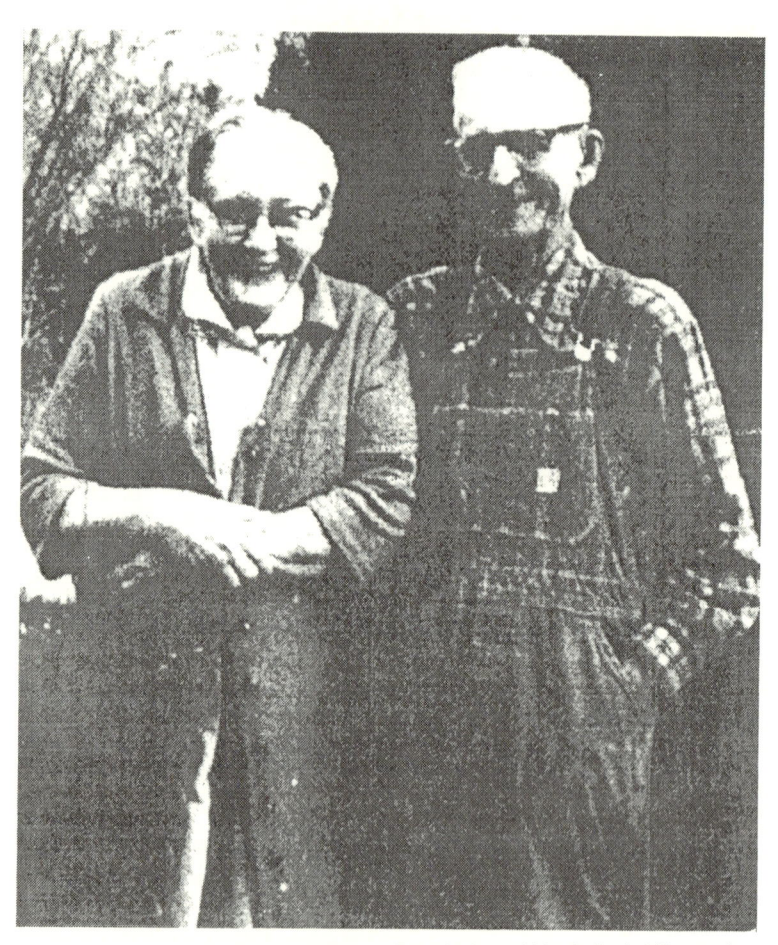

Smiling Etta "Granny" Nichols of Del Rio, who died on Friday, is shown with her husband of 67 years, James Harrison Nichols. She picked up the profession of midwifery from her father and grandfather, who together practiced medicine in Cocke County for more than 80 years. This award-winning photograph was taken by the Nichols' postman.

Wednesday, November 30, 1994

Our Opinion

Etta Nichols brought new life to community

The passing of Etta Nichols represents more than the death of a remarkable woman; it signals the passing of an era in our history.

In today's world, Etta Nichols would never have gotten very far in life. She received no education beyond the eighth grade and certainly would have very few prospects in this on-line world of internets.

But Etta Nichols had the good luck, to be born into a time when what you were was not measured by how far you went in school, it was determined by, as Dr. Martin Luther King said, "the content of your character."

And Etta Nichols had plenty of character to go around. The daughter and granddaughter of men with medical training, she set her heart on being a nurse and delivering babies. So, in the style of the times, she went out and did it. She took no long college courses, passed no tests for certification, applied for jobs at no hospitals or Health Management Organizations, she just went out and delivered babies.

And she learned how to deliver babies not by watching videos, she did it by helping her father and grandfather deliver them. She would even make housecalls to the expectant mothers until it got too difficult for her to get around the mountains of her home.

She never charged more than $15 for a delivery and never asked a mother the name of her co-payer. For she was motivated not by money, but by service to others.

It is certain that, given a choice, a lot of us would not mind taking an extended vacation to a time when things were not quite so organized and time seemed to pass just a little bit slower.

Good-bye Etta Nichols; and farewell to a kinder and gentler time.

(News articles and photos, courtesy of The Newport Plain Talk)

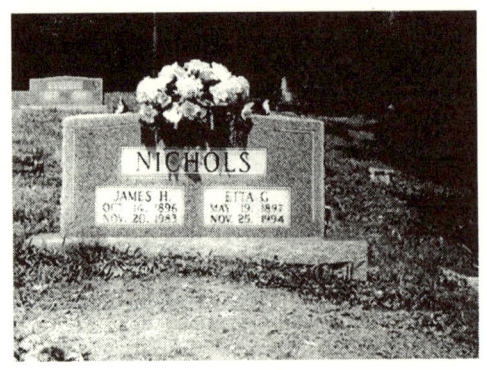

A TRIBUTE
published in the pages of
THE MOUNTAIN PRESS
SEVIERVILLE, TN
NOV 2 6 1994

Memorial Obituary

*Entered Into Eternal Rest
Friday, Nov. 25, 1994*

Etta "Granny" Nichols

Etta "Granny" Nichols, 97, of Del Rio, died Friday at the home of her daughter, Mrs. Floyd Smith of Del Rio.

She was a member of Bridgeport Free Will Baptist Church. She was preceded in death by her husband, James Harrison Nichols, her daughter, Emily Jones, two grandchildren and one great-grandchild.

Survivors include her children, June Gilliland of Morristown, Jack Nichols and Belle Smith of Del Rio; 12 grandchildren; 27 great-grandchildren; seven great-great grandchildren; her sister, Alverta Taylor of Jacksonville, Fla.; and her brother, Furman Grigsby of Bridgeport.

Funeral services will be held at 8 p.m. Sunday at the Brown Funeral Home Chapel with the Rev. Robert Ashley officiating. The family will receive friends from 6 to 8 p.m. prior to the service. Burial will be at 10 a.m. Monday in the Jones Town Cemetery. The Brown Funeral Home in Newport is in charge.

Pallbearers will be great-grandsons, David Gilbert, Darren Burgin, Dusty Brooks, Terry Wall, Johnny Wall and Russell Smith.

Mary,
God Bless You
Sharon Smith-Ledford

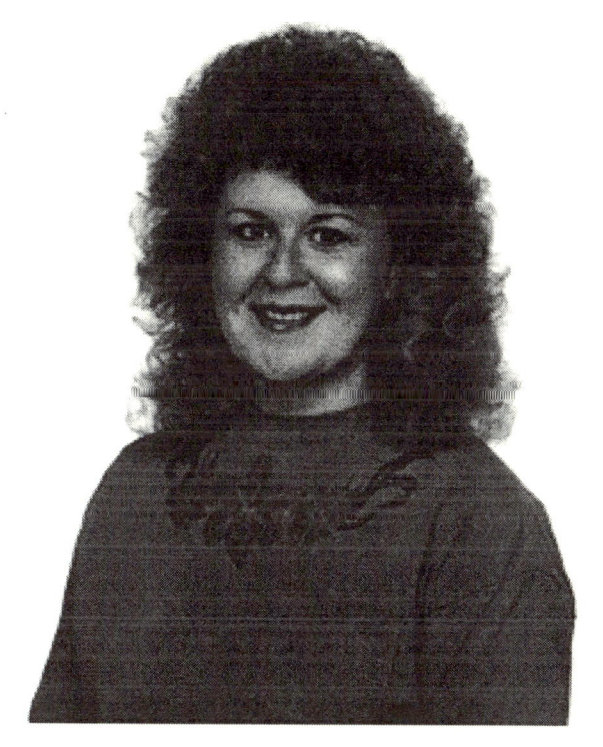

Born in 1957, Sharon Kay Smith-Ledford is the fourth child of Mr. and Mrs. Floyd J. Smith. She was raised about a mile away from her grandmother, Etta Nichols. She attended Del Rio Elementary School, and Cocke County High School. After graduating in 1974, Sharon attended Morristown Voc/Tech where she studied Office Occupations. From there she went on to Walter's State Community College. Sharon now lives in Morristown, Tennessee with her husband, Calvin T. Ledford, and her daughter, Tiffany Alise Smith. Sharon is the back office manager for College Square Travel Agency.

To order additional copies of ETTA "GRANNY" NICHOLS—LAST OF THE OLD-TIMEY MIDWIVES, complete the information below (please print):

NAME_____
ADDRESS_____
CITY, STATE, ZIP_____
PHONE_____

Please send me _____ copies of
Etta "Granny" Nichols—Last of the
Old-Timey Midwives @ $15.00 each
(soft cover only) . . . . Total Price_____

S&H, $4.95 ea. book   Total
                          Shipping & Handling_____

Tennessee residents
add 8.5% sales tax   Total Tax_____

                    Total Amount Enclosed_____

For payments made with personal checks, please allow 4-6 weeks for delivery. For immediate delivery, send cashier check, or money order to:

  Sharon S. Ledford
  P. O. Box 3412
  Morristown, TN 37815-3412

THANK YOU SO MUCH FOR YOUR ORDER!